an outline of
psychiatry

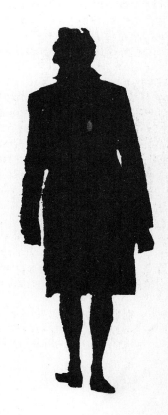

seventh edition
an outline of
psychiatry
Clarence J. Rowe, M.D.
St. Paul, Minnesota

Clinical Professor of Psychiatry
College of Medical Sciences
University of Minnesota, Minneapolis

Psychiatric Consultant
Constance Bultman Wilson Center
Faribault, Minnesota

Psychiatric Consultant
Ramsey County Court System
St. Paul, Minnesota

Medical Director
Adult Psychiatric Service
United Hospitals
St. Paul, Minnesota

In collaboration with Shirley H. Mink, Ph.D
and Walter D. Mink, Ph.D

wcb
Wm. C. Brown Company Publishers
Dubuque, Iowa

wcb

Wm. C. Brown, Chairman of the Board
Larry W. Brown, President, WCB Group

Book Team

Susan J. Soley, Editor
Joyce S. Oberhausen, Production Editor
Marla A. Schafer, Designer

Wm. C. Brown Company Publishers, College Division

Lawrence E. Cremer, President
Raymond C. Deveaux, Vice President/ Product Development
David Wm. Smith, Assistant Vice President/National Sales Manager
Matt Coghlan, National Marketing Manager
David A. Corona, Director of Production Development and Design
William A. Moss, Production Editorial Manager
Marilyn A. Phelps, Manager of Design
Mary M. Heller, Visual Research Manager

To my family
  Patricia
  Padraic
  Rory and
  Kelly Michael

Who persevered through it all

And to
  Burtrum C. Schiele, M.D.

Who showed me the way

Innocens non timidus

Contents

Introduction to the Seventh Edition

Psychiatric practice has changed a great deal in the twenty-six years this Outline has been in print. In each successive edition, I have tried to reflect the changes. The book, originally intended to make psychiatry understandable to students of nursing, physical therapy, and occupational therapy, as well as to other paramedics, has enjoyed wider acceptance with each subsequent edition. In this edition, an attempt has been made to present general areas of clinical psychiatry in outline form. Again, as in the past, no claim to uniqueness is made. The contents reflect my clinical experience in teaching, consulting, and practice. Everything contained here can be found in more elaborate form in the standard textbooks on psychiatry, many of which are listed as references at the ends of the chapters.

Our classification of mental disorders follows the American Psychiatric Association's *Diagnostic and Statistical Manual of Mental Disorders, Third Edition (DSM-III)*. At the time of publication of this *Outline*, the final edition of *DSM*-III was still in press. However, the *Outline* is consonant with all published material on the *DSM*-III and also with material presented at a conference entitled "*DSM*-III: Psychiatric Diagnosis for the 1980s," which was chaired by Robert L. Spitzer, M.D. (the APA task force chairman) in New York City December 6, 7, and 8, 1979. Thus there may be a few minor but not substantive changes in the final edition of *DSM*-III. It should be kept in mind that the *DSM*-III is offered as a *guideline* for clinical psychiatrists. As stated in its Foreword, "the purpose of *DSM*-III is to provide clear descriptions of diagnostic categories to enable clinicians and research investigators to diagnose, treat, study, and communicate about the various mental disorders. It attempts to describe comprehensively *what* is wrong in the mental disorders; it does not attempt to account for *how* the disturbances come about, unless the mechanism is inherent in the definition of the disorder."

Several organizing principles have been used in *DSM*-III to determine the grouping of individual disorders into classes. In order of priority, they are as follows. (1) Known necessary organic etiology. This constitutes the foundation for the classes of Organic Mental Disorders and Substance Use Disorders. (2) Shared phenomenology. This principle includes both the cross-sectional clinical picture and the longitudinal course of a disorder, and is the basis for the class that includes Schizophrenic Disorders, Paranoid Disorders, Schizoaffective Disorders, Affective Disorders, Anxiety Disorders, Somatoform Disorders, Dissociative Disorders, Personality Disorders, and Disorders of Impulse Control. (3) Known or presumed necessary psychosocial etiology. This is the basis for the class of Reactive Disorders Not Elsewhere Classified, and includes the Adjustment Disorders. Neuroses, a traditional category, has been eliminated because "intrapsychic conflict exists in so many psychiatric disorders as well as in persons without psychiatric disorders."

The new nomenclature follows a multiaxial classification. Five axes have been chosen. These five are Axis I: Clinical Psychiatric Syndrome(s) and Other Conditions; Axis II: Personality Disorders (adults) and Specific Developmental Disorders (children and adolescents), see chapter, "Personality Disorders," page 117; Axis III: Physical Disorders, see chapter, "Psychological Factors Affecting Physical Condition (Psychophysiologic Disorders)," page 105; Axis IV: Severity of Psychosocial Stressors, and Axis V: Highest Level of Adaptive Functioning Past Year.

A Psychiatric Glossary, Fifth Edition (Washington, D.C.: American Psychiatric Association, 1980), has helped me formulate some of the definitions.

A special word of thanks is due my colleagues, David E. Schalker, M.D. and Charles C. McCafferty, M.D., for their patience in reviewing most of the manuscript and for their helpful criticisms and suggestions. I am grateful to Dr. Shirley H. Mink and Dr. Walter D. Mink for their many critical comments and their written contributions to the manuscript, signed and unsigned. Sharon Weitzel, a steering committee of one, patiently guided the manuscript to completion.

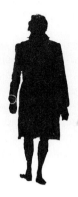

The mind of men is a mystery; and, like the plant, each one of us naturally appropriates and assimilates that about him which responds to that which is within him.

Joseph Roux:
"Prelude," *Meditations of a Parish Priest* (1886)

Etiology of Mental Disorders

I. Introduction

A. Definition

Webster's Third New International Dictionary (1971) defines etiology as—

1. A science or doctrine of causation or the demonstration of causes.
2. A branch of science dealing with the causes of particular phenomena.
3. All the factors that contribute to the occurrence of a disease or abnormal condition; cause; origin.

B. Actually, the essential causes of many mental disorders are unknown or incompletely understood. It is thus necessary for us to consider all the factors that could play a role in the development of any particular mental disorder.

C. One view is that mental disorder results from the interaction of the person (personality) with predisposing and precipitating factors. Subsumed in this view are the following:

1. Predisposing factors are those that render the personality susceptible or vulnerable and are present over a long period of time (subclinical).
2. Precipitating factors are events that precede the clinical onset of the disorder.
3. The severity of the predisposing factors determines the person's vulnerability or susceptibility to precipitating factors.
4. Precipitating factors of varying severity may produce disorder in mildly predisposed persons. For example:
   a. A loosely disorganized schizophrenic may be inordinately upset by a mild social rebuff.
   b. A well-integrated person may develop a mild anxiety reaction to a catastrophe, such as a fire or a flood.
5. Predisposing factors endure throughout the life of the individual. They may be cumulative or connected. Precipitating factors occur intermittently throughout the individual's lifetime. They may be related to special developmental tasks (see p. 5).

D. As a matter of fact, human behavior at any time is determined by the individual's mental status and his or her capacity, at that moment, to adapt to the immediate environment.

E. In the past, two major hypotheses have been advanced to account for mental illness: the psychogenic theory and the somatogenic theory.

1. Proponents of *psychogenic hypothesis* regard mental disorder as an inefficient and unsuccessful compromise to the conflict between the demands of the real world and the individual's desires.
2. Proponents of *somatogenic hypothesis* regard mental illness as resulting from the malfunction of the central nervous system. Such malfunction may be genetically transmitted.

F. The psychogenic and somatogenic hypotheses have been viewed as conflicting alternatives. This view is unnecessarily dualistic. All factors interact, whether they are categorized as "psychosocial" or "organic." It is the *interaction* of the factors that must be considered in any etiology.

G. One way of ranking factors is to separate those that contribute to vulnerability or susceptibility to stress (predisposing) from those that are stressors (the precipitating factors or psychosocial stressors as listed in *DSM*-III). A partial listing of predisposing factors and precipitating factors that are frequently considered in etiological studies is contained in the following sections.

II. Predisposing factors

A. Vulnerability

Vulnerability is a function of predisposing factors, which include the following:

1. Genetics

a. In the diasthesis-stress theory it is assumed that certain genes or combinations of genes give rise to a predisposition (diasthesis) to a particular disorder, which will then be manifested as a result of certain kinds of environmental stress. There is some evidence to support this theory:

(1) The incidence of schizophrenic disorders is much higher in the offspring of schizophrenics than in the general population. The onset of the illness might be related to a particular stress during the person's development.

(2) The incidence of bi-polar disorder (previously called manic-depressive disease) is higher among the offspring of bi-polar depressive parents than in the general population.

(3) Many kinds of dementia (organic loss of intellectual function) seem to be hereditary. Two are noted below.

(a) Huntington's chorea (a degenerative disease of the basal ganglia and cerebral cortex).

(b) Porphyria (an episodic metabolic disorder characterized by the excretion of porphyrins in the urine and accompanied by attacks of abdominal pain, peripheral neuropathy, and a variety of mental symptoms).

b. However, it should be kept in mind that pathological emotional states may be transmitted by parents to their offspring by the parents' deviant behavior rather than through the germ plasm. Such illnesses are familial rather than hereditary.

2. Age
    a. Certain periods of life are considered periods of special stress, not only because of the physical changes that occur but also because of specific psychological stresses that are encountered during such periods.
    b. Adolescence, middle life (sometimes called the involutional period), and the senium (the geriatric age, the period of old age) are many times thought of as periods of special stress.

B. Gender
1. More women than men with emotional problems consult physicians.
2. Affective disorders are more common among women.
3. Alcoholism is much more frequent among men.
4. More attempts at suicide are made by women in the United States, but more men are successful.

III. Precipitating factors
A. Environment

Environment includes the emotional as well as the physical milieu. Among environmental factors are the following:
1. Various family interactions (engagement, marriage, discord, separation, death, becoming a parent, conflict with a child, illness in a child)
2. Other interpersonal relationships (difficulties with friends, neighbors, or associates)
3. Living circumstances (change in residence, immigration)
4. Financial affairs (inadequate finances, financial reverses)
5. Legal affairs (being arrested, suing, being sued)
6. Occupation (conflict with a supervisor, competition for promotion, but *not* overwork, which is usually a symptom rather than a cause of an emotional problem).

B. Physical illness

Physical illness may pose both practical and emotional problems. Among these are the following:
1. Personal (pain, discomfort, enforced idleness).
2. Financial (cost of treatment, inability to make a living).
3. Emotional (reactivation of repressed conflicts, especially those related to feelings of dependency).
4. Body image (mutilative surgery, e.g., breast amputation, may cause certain disturbances of body image).
5. Endocrinal (e.g., hyperthyroidism may lead to tension and anxiety; hypothyroidism may lead to apathy and lethargy).

C. Physical handicaps

Physical handicaps may or may not give rise to emotional disturbances.

1. They may serve as a focus of inferiority feelings and result in such undesirable defenses as overcompensation (see chapter, "Adaptations to Anxiety").
2. However, many persons with physical handicaps do not manifest any significant emotional problems.

D. Exogenous factors

Exogenous factors include drugs, chemicals, infections, and trauma.

1. Drugs and chemicals (alcohol, sedatives, narcotics, and industrial toxins, for example) cause organic mental disorder, or organic brain syndrome, or otherwise affect the individual's adaptive response.
2. Certain infectious diseases may lead to delirium. Syphilis may produce changes in the central nervous system with or without mental disease.
3. Trauma may lead to reversible or irreversible changes, with accompanying personality disorders, or to post-traumatic disorders.

E. Deprivations and deficiencies

1. Starvation, for example, may lead to personality changes (meanness, suspiciousness, withdrawal).
2. Sensory deprivation, of sight, for example, may lead to delirium with hallucinations (following cataract extraction when the eyes are kept covered postoperatively or the hallucinations described by lone explorers or sailors).
3. Deprivation of sleep may lead to mental and personality changes (inability to concentrate, restlessness, apathy).

IV. **Stages in development**

A. Although development is a continuum, it is often divided into stages for convenience of description and discussion.
B. The developmental stages can serve as a background against which to consider any developmental sources of stresses and tasks whose resolution may contribute to vulnerability.
C. Following is an outline of Erik Erikson's psychosocial stages of life as elaborated by Lawrence R. Allman and Dennis T. Jaffee.*

*Abridged and adapted from Table 2.1 "Expanded outline of Erik Erikson's psychosocial stages of life" (p. 32) in *Abnormal Psychology in the Life Cycle* by Lawrence R. Allman and Dennis T. Jaffe. General Editor Phillip Whitten. Copyright © 1978 by Lawrence R. Allman and Dennis T. Jaffe and Phillip Whitten. By permission of Harper & Row, Publishers, Inc.

Life State	Approximate Age Period	Developmental Tasks
Infancy	0 – 2	Social attachment; object permanence; sensorimotor intelligence; maturation of motor functions
Toddlerhood	2 – 4	Self-control; language development; fantasy and play
Early childhood	5 – 7	Sex role identification; early moral development; group play
Middle childhood	8 – 12	Social cooperation; self-evaluation; skill learning; team play
Early adolescence	13 – 17	Peer group membership; heterosexual relationships
Later adolescence	18 – 22	Autonomy from parents; sex role identity; career choice values
Early adulthood	23 – 30	Marriage, childbearing, work, life style
Middle adulthood	31 – 40	Management of household and career; child raising
Middle life	40 – 55	Coming to terms with achievements; career revision; consolidation of identity.
Aging	55 +	Redirection of energy to diminishing role; perspective of death; acceptance of own life

V. Etiology of mental disorders

A. The etiology of emotional disorders should be regarded as a complex and complicated interaction of genetic, psychosocial, and physical factors.

   1. Some of these factors are probably inborn, some develop so early that they become an integral part of the "basic" personality structure, and others come into play later on.

   2. These statements can be represented schematically, but first let us define our terms again.

      a. Hereditary factors include the presence or absence of mental disorder in the family, the innate capacity to cope, physical endowment, etc.

      b. Early environmental influences include parental attitudes, family interaction, and sociocultural factors.

      c. Well-developed defenses (see chapter on adjustive patterns).

d. Stress (physical trauma, loss of love object).

e. Mental disorder (e.g., anxiety, affective disorder, various psychotic disorders).

3. Thus, hereditary factors + early environmental influences (lead to) → the production of well-developed defenses + subsequent stress (may lead to) → mental disorder.

B. Therefore, mental disorders may result from the interaction of predisposing and precipitating factors with the personality.

References

American Psychiatric Association. *Diagnostic and Statistical Manual of Mental Disorders,* 3d ed., Washington, D.C., 1979.

Bosselman, B. *Neurosis and Psychosis.* 3d ed. Springfield, Ill.: Charles C Thomas, 1969, chap. 1.

Kolb, L. C. *Modern Clinical Psychiatry,* 9th ed. Philadelphia: W. B. Saunders Company, 1977, chap. 7.

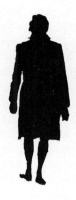

There is occasions and causes why
and wherefore in all things.

Shakespeare: *King Henry V*

Psychodynamic
Concepts

I. Introduction

A. Physical development

The human organism undergoes a process of physical development from the moment of conception (fusion of sperm with ovum) until it reaches maturity. In part, this process is influenced by genetic determinants, but it also is affected by subsequent forces that may impair its goal, produce malfunctions, or limit the functioning of all or part of the organism. These forces derive largely from the experience of the organism in the environment.

B. Psychological development

Similarly, the same person undergoes a process of psychological development (maturation) that is also influenced by hereditary background and various environmental influences. Included in the latter are parental relationships, peer relationships, and cultural and social experiences.

II. Personality development

A. Personality

1. Personality has been defined in various ways. Simply stated, personality is the sum total of the individual's internal and external patterns of adjustment to life.
2. Personality is, in part, determined by one's genetically transmitted organic endowment and in part by one's life experiences.
3. As the individual develops, his or her behavior also changes. Thus, a newborn reacts differently to a given environmental stimulus than an adolescent or adult.
4. For the various stages of personality development, see page 5.

B. In this chapter, we cover various conceptions of human behavior and its motivation.

III. Psychodynamic concepts

A. Definition

Psychodynamics is the study, explanation, or interpretation of behavior or mental states in terms of mental or emotional forces or processes.

B. History

1. Sigmund Freud

Most of our current conceptions of behavioral development and psychopathology originated with the work of Sigmund Freud, who created psychoanalytic theory and therapy. His account of unconscious mental processes has had a profound effect on our society and science.

2. Earlier theorists

Actually, degrees of consciousness were recognized before Freud.

a. Gottfried Wilhelm Liebniz (1646–1716), the German philosopher and mathematician, believed that perception of elements occurred unconsciously.

b. Johann Friedrich Herbart (1776–1841) developed the dynamic theory of unconscious mental functions.

c. Gustav Theodor Fechner (1801–1887) referred to "negative sensations" that occurred below the threshold of consciousness.

d. Hermann Helmholtz (1821–1894) coined the term "unconscious inference."

e. Eduard von Hartman (Karl Robert) (1842–1906), was a metaphysical philosopher who was called "the philosopher of the unconscious."

C. The term *psychoanalysis* has two meanings:

1. A collection of data, based on observations, that led to a theory of abnormal behavior as well as to a general theory of normal personality development

2. The name of a psychotherapeutic technique.

D. A comprehensive résumé of psychoanalytic theories is beyond the scope of this Outline. However, a few of the basic psychoanalytic concepts that have been found useful in general psychiatry will be listed.

IV. Sigmund Freud (1856–1939)

A. Thinking

Freud viewed thinking as composed of primary and secondary processes. This differentiation is viewed by many of his followers as his greatest accomplishment.

1. Primary processes

The psychological expressions of the underlying basic drives. They are assumed to be largely unconscious, present at birth, and thus can be considered innate. They are the more primitive modes of thinking. They are manifested in dreams but are also present during waking life. Thinking at this level follows the *pleasure principle*—the seeking of pleasure and the avoidance of pain.

2. Secondary processes

These are the reasonable and acceptable ways in which the underlying basic drives are controlled and permitted expression according to the demands of the outside world. They are characteristic modes of preconscious and conscious thinking and follow the *reality principle*.

B. Drives

There are certain significant desires and drives that are repressed. These constitute the *dynamic unconscious,* and they resist conscious expression because of their basic unacceptability (see "repression" in the chapter, "Adaptations to Anxiety").

C. Resistance

An individual resists attempts to make these repressed forces conscious through the use of defenses (see "Adaptations to Anxiety"). This constitutes what Freud called *resistance*.

D. Transference

Transference is the displacement of feelings for significant people in one's earlier life onto the physician or therapist.

E. Mind

To help explain all of these phenomena, Freud postulated a mind composed of the conscious, the preconscious (foreconscious), and the unconscious.

1. *The conscious* is composed of ideas, feelings, drives, and urges of which the person is aware. It is the scene of purposeful behavior.

2. *The preconscious,* which is midway between the conscious and the unconscious, comprises feelings, ideas, drives, and urges that are out of the individual's continuous awareness but that can be readily recalled. For example, you may not think about what you ate for supper last night, but you could easily recall the menu if asked.

3. *The unconscious* is made up of drives, feelings, ideas, and urges that are outside of the individual's awareness. One does not acknowledge or label them.

F. Divisions of personality

Psychoanatomically (structurally), Freud divided personality into three parts:

1. Id

The *id* is the unconscious reservoir of primitive drives (instincts). The id is dominated by the primary process manner of thinking and the pleasure principle. It exists in all humans and in modified forms in all other animal life. Components of the id are:

a. *Eros* is the name Freud gave to the creative forces, the life instinct. (Eros was the Greek god of love and originally represented the primeval power that created order and cohesion out of chaos.)

b. *Thanatos* is Freud's term for the aggressive, destructive, or death forces. (Thanatos was the Greek god who personified death and the twin brother of Hypnos, or sleep.)

c. *Homeostasis* is the individual's tendency to maintain a relatively stable psychological condition with respect to contending drives, motivations, and other psychodynamic forces. Freud felt that psychological growth depended on a proper balance between the creative and aggressive forces, with somewhat of a preponderance of the former.

d. *Libido* is Freud's term for the emotional energy broadly derived from these underlying instincts (psychosexual energy) and presumably present at birth. The id serves as a reservoir for the libido, which has two general forms.

    (1) *Ego libido* is libido concentrated on the self, or narcissism. *Primary narcissism* is the original state of the newborn. (Narcissus was a Greek youth who fell in love with his own reflection in the water.)

    (2) *Object libido* is libido that is directed outward toward another person or thing.

e. *Cathexis* is the name Freud gave to the process by which the unconscious primitive drives are vested with psychic energy.

2. Ego

The *ego* is the part of the personality that meets and interacts with the outside world; the "integrator" or "mediator" of the personality.

a. The ego functions to help the individual deal with the world and yet to satisfy the underlying needs of the id through coping and problem-solving (see "Adaptations to Anxiety").

b. It functions at all three levels of consciousness (conscious, preconscious, and unconscious).

c. The adaptive functions of the ego are the defenses against anxiety (see "Adaptations to Anxiety").

d. The opposition of ego energy to id energy is called *counter-cathexis*.

e. The ego is the executive function of the personality.

3. Superego

The superego is the censoring force of the personality. It is composed of the morals, mores, values, and ethics of the individual and is largely derived from one's parents.

a. The conscious part of the superego is called *conscience,* but it operates at all three levels of consciousness.

b. Most of us are conscious of our moral and ethical beliefs but remember only a portion of the training and experience that contributed to the formation of those beliefs.

c. If the ego contemplates violation of the superego's code, anxiety results; if the person carries out the contemplated violation despite the anxiety, guilt feelings ensue.

d. The infant's superego is primitive and undeveloped. It begins to develop in the second year and takes definite form at the age of four or five.

e. The punitive aspect of superego concerns itself with prohibitions, self-criticism, and guilt feelings (bad conscience).

f. The nonpunitive, positive aspect of the superego is sometimes separately designated as the *ego-ideal.*

g. An overly strict superego usually leads to the development
of a rigid, compulsive, unhappy person. A weak, defective
superego permits a person to express hostile and antisocial
strivings without anxiety or guilt.

G. Libido development (stages of psychosexual development)
Freud believed that the major development of adult personality
takes place in infancy and early childhood.

1. The oral phase
   a. The first twelve to eighteen months of life are characterized
   chiefly by preoccupation with feeding. Pleasure is derived
   mainly through the mouth. This period is called *the oral
   phase.*

   b. The early part of the oral phase, *the sucking stage,* is passive.

   c. The later oral phase, or *biting stage,* is aggressive (oral-
   sadistic).

2. The anal phase
   a. From the eighteenth month until the end of the third year,
   the infant's attention is centered on excretory functions.
   This is *the anal phase.*

   b. This is the first time the infant must adjust his or her
   behavior to the demands of others.

   c. This stage is also the foundation for the development of the
   superego.

   d. *Expulsive and retentive phases* are part of the anal phase,
   just as passive and aggressive ones are part of the oral
   phase.

3. The narcissistic or pregenital phase
   The oral and anal phases considered together are called *the
   narcissistic or pregenital phase* because the child's libido is
   satisfied within his or her own body.

4. The phallic phase
   The *phallic phase* extends from the end of the third year to
   the seventh year. The child becomes aware of his or her genitalia. During this stage, for the first time, the child's libido is
   directed outward and requires others for its satisfaction. It is
   characterized, psychosexually, by:

   a. *Castration anxiety,* which results from the boy's fear of
   damage to or loss of his genitals. It includes the childhood
   fantasy that female genitals result from the loss of the
   penis.

b. *Penis envy* is the girl's desire to possess a penis and, thus, to become masculine.

c. *The Oedipus complex* is the attachment of the child to the parent of the opposite sex, accompanied by envious and aggressive feelings toward the parent of the same sex.

    (1) This complex of aggressive feelings in the girl is called the *Electra complex.*

    (2) The resolution of this complex is usually accomplished by subsequent identification with the parent of the same sex.

5. Latency

Latency is the stage between the Oedipal period and the adolescent years. In general, during this period, the person learns to recognize and cope with reality.

6. The genital phase

The *genital phase* is the final stage of psychosexual development.

a. It begins with puberty, with the physiological capacity for orgasms as well as the capacity for object love and mature heterosexuality.

b. The early adolescent stage is narcissistic in that selfish interests predominate.

c. Following this, there is a temporary homosexual phase in which adolescents prefer to meet in gatherings of the same sex.

d. As adolescence progresses, attraction to the opposite sex begins to assert itself more strongly and the capacity for object love and mature heterosexuality emerges.

V. Alfred Adler (1870–1937).

A. Individual psychology

Adler founded the school of *individual psychology*—each person has his or her own special goals and unique manner of achieving them.

B. Organ inferiority

Adler placed more emphasis on the ego than on sexuality.

1. He regarded organ inferiority as the most important etiological factor.

2. He believed that the individual's development was determined by the adaptive push for superiority, or the drive to power. (The specific type of superiority depends upon the individual's biological background and early environment.)

3. In this quest for power, a particular *life-style*—the individual's step-wise, active, unique adaptation to the social milieu—evolves.

C. Personality

Adler regarded personality as developing out of the individual's attitudes toward herself or himself, toward other people (especially family), and toward society.

D. Inferiority complex

1. Adler coined the term *inferiority complex* to describe the conflict, partly conscious and partly unconscious, that impels the individual to attempt to overcome the distress accompanying feelings of inferiority (which are derived from the helplessness of the infant).

2. He believed that a neurotic disposition is caused by overprotection, neglect, or both, during childhood.

3. The person with strong feelings of inferiority may, however, compensate by trying to become superior in some special area.

4. The struggle for superiority may be successful, if modified by the demands of reality.

5. Thus, in the Adlerian formulation, neurosis represents the various psychological processes by which the individual seeks to cope with his or her inferiority.

E. Masculine protest

1. *Masculine protest* is Adler's term for the individual's attempt to escape from the feminine, submissive role. Women become tomboys or tyrannical mothers or wives. Men become Don Juans.

2. Masculine protest may derive from the subject's own uncertainty of his or her role.

VI. **Carl G. Jung** (1871–1961)

A. Analytic psychology

Jung's modification of psychoanalysis was called *analytic psychology*.

B. Introversion and extroversion

Jung stressed life goals and the role of introversion and extroversion in personality development.

1. He defined *introversion* as inwardly directed libido, reflected in the tendency to be preoccupied with oneself.

2. *Extroversion* was his term for outwardly directed libido.

C. The libido

1. Like Adler, Jung minimized the role of sexuality in personality dynamics.

2. He believed that the libido was broadly derived from all life energy (not just from sex).

D. The unconscious

1. In addition to the *personal* unconscious, Jung postulated a *collective* unconscious (racial or archaic unconscious), believing that there was an inheritance of primitive racial ideas and impulses.

2. He believed the personal unconscious to be superficial and hence more accessible then the collective unconscious.
3. The collective unconscious was later called the *objective psyche*. It included both—
   a. *Autochthonous ideas,* ideas originating within the psyche without external stimuli.
   b. *Primordial images,* a phylogenetic memory heavily laden with mythological reference.
E. The persona and anima
   1. The *persona* is the social facade assumed by an individual (so named from the mask worn by actors in ancient Greek drama, which characterized the mood portrayed). The individual behaves in conformity with what is expected of him or her.
   2. The *anima* is the true inner self, or soul. In addition,
      a. The *animus* is the masculine component of the female personality.
      b. The *anima* is the female component of the male personality.
F. Basic psychological functions
   1. Adler described four basic psychological functions: (1) feelings, (2) thinking, (3) sensation, and (4) intuition. (The first two are usually conscious; the second two are usually unconscious.)
   2. In addition, he saw people as having two general attitudes: (1) extroversion, and (2) introversion.
   3. Thus, there were eight possible combinations.
G. Therapy
   Jung believed that psychiatric treatment should deal with current problems and plans for the future as well as attempts to uncover past causal experiences.

VII. **Otto Rank** (1884–1939)
A. The birth trauma.
   Rank proffered the theory that *the birth trauma* was central to the individual's experience.
   1. The process of birth produces primal anxiety in response to feelings of helplessness.
   2. Separation from the mother is the original trauma, a sudden, violent change from the security of intrauterine existence to the uncertainties of the outer world.
   3. Subsequent separations of any type are also traumatic.
   4. Every pleasure is a seeking of the reestablishment of intrauterine primal pleasure.
B. Conflict and therapy
   1. As the child becomes conscious of himself as separate from his mother, he develops conflict.
   2. The desire for separation leads to guilt feelings.

3. According to Rank, a person has difficulty asserting his or her will.
4. In adulthood, a person possesses "a good" portion (approved by his parents and society), and a "bad" portion, called *counterwill* (which is disapproved).
5. Relieving guilt feelings is the central focus of treatment.

C. Personality
Rank described three character types:
1. The normal or average person (who accepts the will of the group)
2. The creative person (who sets his or her own ideals and governs himself or herself accordingly)
3. The neurotic person (who is not free to express his or her own will, but cannot conform to the group).

VIII. Karen Horney (1885–1952)

A. The social and emotional environment
Karen Horney focused on the dynamics of social and environmental factors in personality development.

B. Sexuality
1. Horney did not accept the Freudian theory of the libido and his emphasis on infantile sexuality.
2. She discounted the theory of penis envy.

C. Anxiety
Horney stressed the principle of basic anxiety.
1. The child's apprehension and insecurity result from relationships with parents who are overindulgent, dominating, erratic, or indifferent.
2. As a consequence, the child is left without a feeling of belonging.
3. Hostility and conflict derive from this basic anxiety.

D. Personality
1. She delineated three main directions a child could take in coping with the environment:
   a. *Moving toward people* (i.e., accepting one's helplessness and attempting to win the affection of others);
   b. *Moving against people* (fighting the surrounding hostility);
   c. *Moving away from people* (remaining apart and neither belonging or fighting).
2. Three types of persons would typify these three basic attitudes:
   a. Compliant
   b. Aggressive
   c. Detached.

E. Self

Central to Horney's theory is the concept of *self,* which could be viewed in three ways—

1. *The actual self* (the sum total of an individual's experiences).
2. *The real self* (the unique total force and sense of integration found in each person).
3. *The idealized self* (a glorified self-image, closely related to the current concept of narcissism), and a sign of neurosis.

F. Therapy

In therapy, she emphasized the self and the environment, concentrating on:

1. Self-realization
2. Self-actualization
3. Dealing with the here-and-now.

IX. Harry Stack Sullivan (1892–1949)

A. Interpersonal theory of psychiatry
1. Harry Stack Sullivan espoused an *interpersonal theory of personality,* i.e., interpersonal relationships provide the experiences that are crucial in personality formation, both normal and abnormal.
2. His views owe something to both psychoanalysis and psychobiology (see "Contributions of Adolf Meyer," p. 21).
3. Social psychiatry has developed from Sullivan's principles.

B. Anxiety
1. Sullivan emphasized the need for security, which he felt could be satisfied only through interpersonal relationships.
2. He conceived of anxiety in the infant as stemming from a disturbance in the relationship between the child and the mothering one.
3. He regarded anxiety as the major factor in personality development as well as in the development of all emotional illnesses and psychopathology.

C. Personality
1. Sullivan believed that personality evolves from the action of personal and social forces in the individual from the time of birth onward.
2. He believed that *the power motive* underlies all other impulses and operates from birth onward to overcome an inner sense of helplessness.
3. He regarded intrapsychic conflicts (from within the personality) as being derived from interpersonal conflicts. That is, they are internalized interpersonal conflicts.

D. Therapy
1. Sullivan believed that treatment must include management of the patient in his or her milieu (environment).

X. Erich Fromm (1900–   )
  A. Alienation
    1. Fromm believes that individuals are a product of their culture and that, in an industrialized society, they have become estranged from their culture and themselves.
  B. Personality
    1. Fromm emphasizes that character is shaped by social and cultural influences and not by internal determinates.
    2. He describes five character patterns:
      a. *Receptive* (depends on others for support)
      b. *Exploitive* (exercises power over others or takes things by guile)
      c. *Marketing* (defines worth in terms of success; regards people as commodities to be bought and sold)
      d. *Hoarding* (possessive; bases security on saving and keeping)
      e. *Productive* (achieves his or her own capacity for love and creative work; has developed fully).
  C. Therapy
    The cultural environment must be considered in the treatment approach.
XI. Erik Erikson (1902–   )
  A. Identity
    1. Erikson emphasizes the concepts of identity (an inner sense of sameness that perseveres, despite external changes), identity crisis, and identity confusion.
    2. His contributions are built upon basic Freudian tenets (in this regard he differs from Jung, Adler, and Horney, who rejected Freud's theories and substituted their own).
    3. Like Adler, he minimized the role of sexuality in personality dynamics.
  B. Psychosocial stages
    Erikson identified eight *psychosocial stages* in personal development (the human life cycle or ego development).
    1. Sensory-oral
      The sensory-oral stage is characterized by trust vs. mistrust (corresponds to Freud's oral stage and usually extends through the first year of life).
    2. Muscular-anal
      The *muscular-anal stage* is characterized by autonomy vs. doubt (corresponds to the anal stage; spans the second and third years of life).
    3. Locomotor-genital
      The *locomotor-genital* stage involves initiative vs. guilt (the genital stage, age four to five).

4. Latency

   Latency involves industry vs. inferiority (age six to eleven; the school age).

5. Puberty and adolscence

   Puberty and adolescence involve ego identity vs. role confusion (roughly, ages twelve to eighteen, when the adolescent is developing a personal identity).

6. Young adulthood

   Young adulthood is characterized by intimacy vs. isolation (roughly, the period of courtship and early family, extending from late adolescence until middle age).

7. Adulthood

   Adulthood is characterized by generativity vs. stagnation or self-absorption (middle age).

8. *Maturity*

   Maturity is characterized by ego integrity vs. despair (the individual's major efforts are nearing completion and there is time for reflection and the enjoyment of any grandchildren).

C. At each stage of development, basic psychosocial crises must be resolved.

XII. Contributions of Adolf Meyer (1866–1950)

A. Psychobiology

1. Adolf Meyer founded *psychobiology* ("psychobiology studies not only the person as a whole, as a unit, but also the whole man").

2. His therapy theory was characterized as distributive analysis and synthesis.

   a. Patients, under the guidance of the therapist, critically evaluate the situations with which they are confronted and their responses to them.

   b. Through discussion and reasoning, the patients try to formulate a way of dealing with their problems more constructively.

3. His was a comprehensive or pluralistic approach to the understanding of mental illness. Thus, he emphasized the need to consider all pertinent information about the life of an individual, as a biological, psychological, and social organism.

4. This is sometimes called *holism,* or the holistic approach (the understanding of the individual personality is based on the interplay of his inherited structure, his uniqueness, and the cultural pattern in which he lives).

5. Despite his holistic approach, he did not focus at all on the family.

6. American psychiatry has been greatly influenced by Meyerian thinking.
7. His approach has relevance to the community mental health movement.
    B. Ego development
       1. He did not systematize his thinking and never outlined developmental stages and their critical tasks.
       2. He spoke of reactions rather than diseases.

XIII. Ego-psychologists
   A. Heinz Hartmann, Ernst Kris, Rudolph Lowenstein.
   B. *Ego psychology* shifted the emphasis from depth psychology to increased emphasis on autonomous or independent functions of the ego (reality testing, control of movement, perception, thinking, etc.).
   C. Described an undifferentiated phase from which both the id and the ego are gradually formed.

XIV. Existential psychoanalysis
   A. Existential psychoanalysis is based on the philosophy of Sartre, Kierkegaard, and others.
   B. This theoretical approach stressed the here-and-now rather than the past in the evaluation of personality disorder.
       1. It is primarily focused on three themes: (1) the person and himself or herself; (2) the person and other persons; and (3) the person and the world he or she lives in.
       2. This theoretical approach has had little influence on present-day psychiatry.

References

Blum, G. S. *Psychodynamics: The Science of Unconscious Mental Forces.* Belmont, Calif.: Brooks/Cole Publishing Company, 1966.

Ewalt, J. R., and Farnsworth, D. L. *Textbook of Psychiatry.* New York: McGraw-Hill Book Company, 1963, chap. 4.

Freedman, A. M.; Kaplan, H. I.; and Sadock, B. J. *Modern Synopsis of Comprehensive Textbook of Psychiatry.* Baltimore: Williams & Wilkins Company, 1976, 2d ed., chaps. 6, 7, and 8.

Kolb, L. C. *Modern Clinical Psychiatry.* 9th ed. Philadelphia: W. B. Saunders Company, 1977, chaps. 2 and 4.

Millon, T. *Theories of Psychopathology.* Philadelphia: W. B. Saunders Company, 1967, part 2.

Nicholi, A. M., Jr., ed.: *The Harvard Guide to Modern Psychiatry.* Cambridge: Belknap Press of Harvard University, 1978, chap. 8.

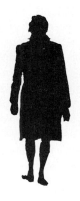

The ideas of goblins and sprights
have really no more to do with
darkness than light; yet let but a
foolish maid inculcate these often on
the mind of a child, . . . possibly he
shall never be able to separate them
again so long as he lives but
darkness shall forever afterward
bring with it those frightful
ideas. . . . Many children imputing
the pain they endured at school to
their books . . . so join those ideas
together that a book becomes their
aversion . . . and thus reading
becomes a torment to them, which
otherwise possibly they might have
made the greatest pleasure of their
lives.

John Locke

Behavioral Concepts: Learning

*by Shirley H. Mink, Ph.D., and
Walter D. Mink, Ph.D.*

I. Introduction

The experimental psychology of learning and learned behavior has been the source of many concepts and techniques that have contributed to the understanding and treatment of psychiatric disorders. In this section, some fundamental concepts about behavior as learned will be introduced. Examples of therapeutic procedures based on these concepts are included in a later chapter, "Treatment in Psychiatry." By way of example, we will cite "token economies" used in institutions for the mentally retarded and the mentally ill, conditioned reflex therapy, desensitization, aversion, and assertiveness training. Behavioral concepts are used and discussed not only by mental health professionals; the roles of reward and punishment in child rearing, individual and social manipulation and control, and free will versus determinism are the subjects of many conversations and debates in the culture at large.

II. Definition

Those who view learning as the basis of psychiatric disorders interpret such disorders as the outcome of experiences in which inappropriate or maladaptive learning, particularly emotional learning, has occurred. A major assumption is that the same principles of learning that account for the development of disordered behavior can be applied in its correction.

III. History

Modern experiments in learning began in Russia with Ivan Pavlov and have continued, primarily in the United States, up to the present.

A. Ivan Pavlov (1849-1936)

Pavlov was a Russian physiologist who discovered classical conditioning during his studies of digestion. He was awarded the Nobel Prize in 1903 for his achievements.

1. The conditioned reflex

Pavlov showed that a reflexive response can, with proper training, be linked to a stimulus that does not normally elicit it.

a. His famous experiments demonstrated that salivation, which occurs reflexively when food is put in the mouth, can also be caused to occur predictably in the presence of a neutral stimulus such as a bell or light.

b. His training procedures involved the presentation of a neutral stimulus (e.g., a bell) slightly before putting food in a dog's mouth. The food caused the dog to salivate. Repeated pairings of the two, bell and food, eventually resulted in salivation when the bell alone was presented.

c. In the standard terminology of classical conditioning, a conditioned stimulus (CS), such as a bell, is repeatedly presented slightly before an unconditioned stimulus (US), such as a piece of food that elicits salivation, an unconditioned reflex or response (UR). The CS will eventually elicit the response, which is then referred to as a conditioned reflex or response (CR).

d. Schematically:

US———→UR
(food)   (salivation)

CS———→CR
(bell)   (salivation)

2. Other phenomena in the conditioning of reflexes
   a. Extinction
      When the CS is repeatedly presented without the US, the CR will decrease and eventually disappear. This phenomenon is called *extinction.*
   b. Generalization
      When a subject has been trained to make a CR in the presence of a CS, the CR tends to occur as a response to stimuli that resemble the original CS. This is known as *generalization.*
   c. Discrimination
      When a subject is trained to respond to the original CS and, during the same training, to ignore stimuli similar to the CS, the subject is said to exhibit *discrimination.*
3. Conditioning of emotional behavior
   Classical conditioning may occur particularly in learned reactions that are mediated by the autonomic nervous system, as is the case with emotional reactions.
4. Experimental neurosis
   a. Pavlov noted a disorganization in the behavior of animals that were required to make extremely difficult conditioned discriminations; he called this phenomenon *experimental neurosis.*
   b. Pavlov applied his analysis to the study of hysteria and obsessional neurosis. His ideas have had a major influence on contemporary Russian psychiatry.

B. Behaviorism
   John B. Watson (1878-1958), an American psychologist, formulated the methodological position in psychology known as *Behaviorism.*
   1. Definition
      a. Watson believed that psychology should be the study of *observable behavior* and should avoid references to unobservable mental functions such as consciousness.
      b. Watson insisted that the experimental study of animal behavior could contribute to the understanding of human behavior and used Pavlov's principles of conditioning to explain human behavior.

2. Watson demonstrated, in 1920, that fears could be induced by classical conditioning.
   a. A one-year-old boy named Albert became fearful of a white rat, which had not frightened him previously, when a loud noise was made behind him while playing with the rat.
   b. After a few trials, Albert became fearful of any white rat *without* the noise, and his fear became *generalized* to other furry animals and objects.
   c. A few years later, Mary Jones replicated Watson's findings and also demonstrated that a conditioned response (fear) could be *eliminated* by conditioning procedures.
C. Operant conditioning
   B. F. Skinner (b. 1904), an American psychologist, refined Watson's methodology and explored what he called operant conditioning. Well known among his important writings are *Walden Two* and *Beyond Freedom and Dignity*.
   1. Definition
      Skinner developed experimental procedures for demonstrating how the consequences of an act influence the subject's tendency to repeat the act. Operant conditioning consists in reinforcing or not reinforcing the consequences of an act so that it tends to be repeated or extinguished. There are several notable features of operant conditioning.
      a. Contingency
         Skinner has shown that the temporal relation of an act to an outcome, such as food or escape from an annoying situation, influences the likelihood that the act will be repeated. The occurrence together of the response and the consequence is called a contingency.
      b. Reinforcement
         In the terminology of operant conditioning, the consequence of a response is called *reinforcement*. The experimental procedure allows the subject (e.g., a rat) to perform a random act (e.g., pressing a lever). If the act results in the delivery of food (a reinforcer), it is said to be reinforced. Repeated pairings of the response and the reinforcement will increase the subject's tendency to press the lever.
         (1) *Positive reinforcement* is the presentation of a reward.
         (2) *Negative reinforcement* is the removal of a noxious or aversive stimulus.
         (3) In either case, the response that produces the changed situation for the subject is the one that is reinforced.
         (4) Stimulus control of a response can also be established by reinforcing the response only in the presence of a particular stimulus, such as a light.

(5) Schematically:

$$S\text{------------}R \longrightarrow S$$

light   press lever   reinforcement (food)

   c. Some other phenomena of operant conditioning
      (1) *Extinction* means that repeated performance of a response in the absence of reinforcement will lead to a decreased occurrence of the response.
      (2) *Punishment* occurs when an aversive or noxious stimulus follows a response. It will suppress (but not extinguish) that response.
      (3) *Discrimination* results when a response to one stimulus, but not to another stimulus, is reinforced. The stimulus that signals the reward becomes a *discriminative stimulus.*
      (4) *Schedules of reinforcement* involve varying the amount of time between reinforcements (*interval schedule*) or the required number of responses between reinforcements (*ratio schedule*). These schedules influence the rate of the response and the resistance to its extinction.
  2. Application of operant conditioning
    a. The principles of operant conditioning have been used to analyze social learning, aggressive behavior, classroom learning, and many other complex forms of behavior.
    b. Many students and collaborators of Skinner have interpreted disordered behavior in operant terms and have developed training procedures for use in hospitals and other institutional settings.
    c. *Autonomic responses*
       Within limits, operant conditioning also affects autonomic responses, as in the self-regulation, through training in biofeedback, of heart rate, blood pressure, and skin temperature.

IV. Behavioral psychology and psychiatry

Many examples of behavioral interpretations of psychiatric concepts can be provided, but those that follow may be sufficient to illustrate the style of behavioral analysis.
  A. Conflict
    1. A behavioral interpretation of conflict stresses the existence of incompatible responses of equal or nearly equal probability.
    2. The most compelling kind of conflict occurs when an *approach response* is elicited by the same situation in which an *avoidance response* is elicited.
    3. An example of an approach-avoidance conflict might be provided by a child who enjoys playing at a neighborhood playground but has been teased there by a bully.

B. Anxiety
   1. Anxiety may be interpreted as a autonomic nervous system reaction that occurs in fearsome or threatening situations but becomes conditioned to irrelevant, coincidental, or unlabeled aspects of the situation (e.g., Albert's fear of the white rat).
   2. Insofar as situations which produce anxiety are aversive, learned ways to escape or avoid the situations may be reinforced.
C. Symptoms
   1. Symptoms are viewed as learned reactions that are the result of previous reinforcement.
   2. If a symptom persists in a situation, then something in the situation is reinforcing it.
   3. Symptoms, just like any other learned response, can be altered by changing the conditions of reinforcement.

References

Hilgard, E. R., and Bower, G. H. *Theories of Learning*, 4th ed. New York: Appleton-Century-Crofts. 1974.

Hoenig, W. K., and Staddon, J. E. R., eds. *Handbook of Operant Behavior*. Englewood Cliffs, N. J.: Prentice-Hall. 1977.

Hulse, S. H.; Deese, J.; and Egeth, H. *The Psychology of Learning*, 4th ed. New York: McGraw-Hill Book Company, 1975.

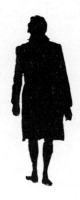

The symptoms of disease are marked by purpose, and the purpose is beneficent. The processes of disease aim not at the destruction of life, but at the saving of it.

Frederick Treves: Address to the Edinburgh Philosophical Institution, October 31, 1905

Symptomatology of Mental Disorders

I. Introduction
   A. Symptoms of mental disorders are expressions of the whole organism, not just the psyche or soma alone.
   B. The manifestations of mental disorders are the result of multiple forces, some of which are extrapsychic (i.e., from the environment) and some of which are intrapsychic (i.e., from within the personality).
   C. Thus, though symptoms may seem perplexing and unusual, they have cause and meaning.
      1. Symptoms represent the patient's effort to maintain his or her emotional equilibrium.
      2. In order to understand their meaning, one must know the patient's life history, including the psychological, sociocultural, and biological needs and the forces that have been of importance in the person's development.
   D. Symptoms of mental disorders are really psychobiological reactions.
II. Somatic symptoms
   Physical symptoms of mental disorders are of three types
   A. Physiological reflections of anxiety:
      Found in the anxiety disorders, including the phobic disorders, obsessive-compulsive disorders, generalized anxiety, and panic.
   B. Symbolic expressions of underlying conflicts
      1. Found in the conversion disorders (symbolic somatization).
      2. Examples are—
         a. Hysterical deafness as a defense against hearing something feared or forbidden.
         b. Hysterical paralysis as a defense against taking action.
   C. Physical symptoms
      Found in other Somatoform Disorders, such as Somatization Disorder (Briquet's Syndrome), Psychogenic Pain Disorder, Hypochondriasis, and Atypical Somatoform Disorder. The essential features of all these disorders are symptoms that suggest physical disorder but for which there is no demonstrable organic basis.
III. Psychological symptoms:
   Psychological symptoms may be manifested in many ways.
   A. Disturbances of affect
      1. Definition
         Affect is mood, feeling, or emotion.
      2. Anxiety
         Anxiety may be defined as uneasiness, apprehension, or fearfulness stemming from anticipated danger, the source of which is unidentifiable. It can be divided into degrees:
         a. *Free-floating anxiety* is severe, persistent, generalized, and unattached anxiety. Typically found in anxiety disorders.

b. *Agitation* is a state of restlessness and uneasiness often characterized by such muscular manifestations as motor restlessness; mental perturbation.

c. *Tension* is tautness, motor and emotional restlessness; dread.

d. *Panic* is an acute anxiety attack of overwhelming severity that leads to disorganization of ego functions. (The word is derived from Pan, the Greek god, who suddenly appeared to unsuspecting travelers in the woods, causing them to "panic").

3. Depression

Depression is a feeling of sadness, loneliness, dejection, or hopelessness, typically found in major depressive disorder and bi-polar depressive disorder. It must be differentiated from *grief,* which is a state of sadness proportionate to a loss.

4. Euphoria

Euphoria is an exaggerated sense of well-being not consistent with reality. Most commonly found in manic disorders and in certain organic mental disorders, including disorders resulting from the use of toxic substances. It may be divided into degrees:

a. *Elation* is marked euphoria accompanied by increased motor activity.

b. *Exultation* is intense elation accompanied by grandiose feelings.

c. *Ecstasy* is a feeling of intense rapture found in states of depersonalization and certain psychoses, such as schizophrenic disorders.

5. Apathy

Apathy is the lack of feeling, emotion, interest, or concern; impassiveness or unfeelingness.

6. Inappropriateness

Inappropriateness is an affect opposite to what would be expected. Observed in schizophrenic disorders, e.g., laughter when a sad message is being expressed.

7. Ambivalence

Ambivalence is the coexistence of two opposing feelings toward the same individual or object; these feelings may be conscious, unconscious, or both. Found in many emotional disorders, but especially in depressive and obsessive-compulsive disorders.

8. Hostility

Hostility is anger, antagonism, opposition, or resistance in thought or behavior. It is the affective counterpart of aggression, to which it is closely allied. It is found in an extreme degree in antisocial personalities and in certain other personality disorders. Unexpressed and internalized hostility is important in the psychodynamics of some depressive disorders.

9. Depersonalization

Depersonalization is a pervasive feeling of unreality, strangeness, or altered identity. Found in depersonalization disorder, schizophrenic disorder, and bi-polar affective illness.

10. Derealization

Derealization is the feeling that the environment has changed. Found in depersonalization disorders and characterized by alternating periods of euphoria or anxiety and depression. Found in cyclothymic disorder (cyclothymic personality).

B. Disturbances of memory

1. Definition

Memory is composed of three processes.

a. *Registration*

The ability to establish a record of an experience in the central nervous system.

b. *Retention*

The persistence or permanence of a registered experience.

c. *Recall*

The ability to recount a registered experience.[1]

2. All of these processes may be disturbed in various ways.

3. Amnesia

Amnesia is a pathological loss of memory. It may be of organic etiology, (e.g., head injury) or psychogenic, as in certain dissociative disorders, (e.g., psychogenic amnesia).

a. *Anterograde amnesia* is loss of memory of events that occur after a particular time.

b. *Retrograde amnesia* is loss of memory of events that occurred before a particular time.

4. Fugue state

A *fugue state* is dissociation, a flight from the immediate environment, characterized by an inability to remember what is happening. The individual escapes from the environment and, during this state, apparently acts purposefully. However, when the person regains consciousness, he or she cannot recall the episode, or fugue. Found in psychomotor equivalents of convulsive disorders and also in the dissociative disorder, psychogenic fugue.

5. Hypermnesia

Hypermnesia is abnormally vivid or complete memory, or the reawakening of impressions long seemingly forgotten. Found both in normal persons and in certain manic and paranoid disorders.

---

1. Adapted from *Modern Synopsis of Comprehensive Textbook of Psychiatry,* vol. 2, ed. A. M. Freedman, H. I. Kaplan, and B. J. Sadock (Baltimore: Williams and Wilkins Co. 1976), p. 392.

6. Paramnesia

Paramnesia is a distortion or falsification of memory in which the individual confuses reality and fantasy. It includes the illusion of remembering scenes and events not experienced before.

    a. *Confabulation* is a falsification of memory in which gaps in memory are filled in by imaginary (fabricated) experiences that seem plausible and are recounted in detail. Found in certain organic mental disorders, especially alcohol amnestic disorder (Korsakoff's syndrome).

    b. *Retrospective falsification* is the unconscious distortion of past experiences to conform to present emotional needs. Found in certain paranoid disorders.

    c. *Fausse reconnaissance* is a false recognition of the unfamiliar.

    d. *Déjà vu* is the sensation that an experience that is really happening for the first time has occurred previously. Occurs to normal people and is found in many mental disorders.

    e. *Jamais vu* is a false feeling of unfamiliarity with a real situation that one has experienced before.

C. Disturbances of consciousness

  1. Definition

    a. Consciousness is synonymous with awareness.

    b. It also means apperception, a mental act in which the mind becomes aware or has knowledge of itself as it perceives.

  2. Both of these aspects of consciousness may be distorted.

  3. Confusion

Confusion is disorientation in respect to time, place, or person and is accompanied by perplexity. Sometimes accompanied by disturbances of consciousness and commonly associated with organic mental disorders.

  4. Clouding of consciousness

Clouding of consciousness is impairment of retention, perception, and orientation. Commonly associated with organic mental disorders, both acute and chronic.

  5. Dream state

Dream state is also known as twilight state. It is a transient clouding of consciousness of intrapsychic origin during which the person is unaware of reality and behaves violently or opposite to his or her usual pattern. Found in dissociative disorders, convulsive disorders, and in association with the use of certain drugs (e.g., Scopoloamine or Atropine-like drugs).

  6. Delirium

Delirium is characterized by disturbance in affect, memory, and consciousness. There are obvious changes in mood, there are illusions, and there are hallucinations. Delirium may be caused by any agent that produces temporary and reversible cerebral metabolic insufficiency, such as alcohol or drugs. Also seen in delirious disorders from acute infectious diseases.

7. Coma

  Coma is stupor, a state of unawareness, nonreactiveness, profound unconsciousness. Found in certain organic mental disorders and in the stuporous form of catatonic schizophrenia.

8. Deterioration

  Deterioration, or dementia, is the progressive loss of intellectual and emotional functions. Found in degenerative diseases of the brain such as Alzheimer's disease, and in primary degenerative dementia. Reversible deterioration is found in schizophrenic disorders.

D. Disturbances of orientation

1. Definition

  Orientation is awareness of one's relationship to time, surroundings, and other persons.

2. Disorientation

  Disorientation is loss of awareness of one's relationship to time, surroundings, or other persons. Usually reversible in certain substance-induced disorders (toxic deliria) and irreversible in chronic mental disorders such as senile and pre-senile dementia.

3. Disorientation in respect to time is the most common, followed by place and person.

E. Disturbances of perception

1. Definition

  Perception is the awareness and intended integration of sensory impressions of the environment and their interpretation in light of experience.

2. Perception may be disturbed or heightened in several ways.

3. Illusions

  Illusions are misinterpretation of sensory experiences, usually optical or auditory. They are frequently normal.

  a. *Optical illusions* are sometimes called mirages as, for example, when heat rays shimmering on a road look like pools of water. Common in acute but reversible substance-induced disorders as, e.g., the withdrawal delirium from alcohol, also known as delirium tremens.

  b. *Auditory illusions* are mistaken interpretations of sounds as, for example, the roaring of the wind heard as the moaning of a human voice.

4. Hallucinations

  Hallucinations are false sensory perceptions that are not caused by external stimuli.

a. They may be auditory, visual, olfactory, gustatory, tactile (haptic), or kinesthetic (phantom limb is a kinesthetic hallucination).
b. Hallucinations occur in substance-use disorders (caused by alcohol, cocaine, or hallucinogenic drugs such as LSD, peyote, or mescaline). May also be found in certain other psychotic conditions such as schizophrenic and manic disorders. Different types of disorders tend to produce different types of hallucinations.
   (1) Colorful or vivid *visual hallucinations* are most typically found in the deliria from acute infectious diseases or in the substance-induced delirious disorders.
   (2) *Auditory hallucinations* are commonly found in schizophrenic disorders.
   (3) *Olfactory hallucinations* occur in schizophrenic disorders and in lesions of the temporal lobe of the brain.
   (4) *Tactile* hallucinations are found in cocaine intoxication and alcohol withdrawal delirium (delirium tremens).
c. An exception to these generalizations about hallucinations is amphetamine-induced organic mental disorder, which commonly produces auditory hallucinations, and sometimes tactile and olfactory ones as well.
d. *Hypnagogic hallucinations* (hypnagogic imagery) are mental images that sometimes occur just before sleep. Images seen in dreams which persist after awakening are called *hypnopompic*. Both types are normal and are familiar to healthy individuals. Hypnogogic states, in particular, are sometimes experienced by persons who are very tired but unable to find the time or place to sleep.

In *Oliver Twist*, Charles Dickens writes: "There is a drowsy state between sleeping and waking when you dream more in five minutes with your eyes half-open and yourself half-conscious of everything that is passing around you, than you would in five nights with your eyes fast closed, and your senses wrapped in perfect consciousness. At such times, a mortal knows just enough of what his mind is doing to form some glimmering conceptions of its mighty powers, its bounding from earth and spurning time and space, when freed from the restraint of its corporeal associate."

Edgar Allan Poe was concerned with such sleepless dreams. In *Marginalia* he writes: ". . . these 'fancies' have in them a pleasurable ecstacy as far beyond the most pleasurable of the world of wakefulness or of dreams, as the Heaven of the Northman theology is beyond its Hell. I regard the visions, even as they arise, with an awe which in some measure moderates or tranquilizes the ecstasy."

5. Eidetic imagery

   Eidetic imagery consists of vivid, accurate, and detailed visual after-images sometimes called photographic memory. Such experiences are normal and are to be distinguished from hallucinations. "Perhaps the artists have a greater eidetic power than most adults," wrote Franz Boaz.

6. Misperceptions

   Misperceptions are associated with conversion disorders (hysterical misperceptions).

   a. Perceptual distortions may occur in any of the sensory areas.
   b. Sensation may be exaggerated or, more commonly, reduced. For example, *hyperesthesia* and *hyperalgesia* or, conversely, *hypesthesia and hypalgesia* may occur in conversion disorder.
   c. *Macropsia* is visualization of objects as larger than they really are, conversely, *micropsia* is visualization of objects as smaller than they really are,

F. Disturbances of thinking

1. Definition

   Thinking is the exercise of powers of judgment, conception, or inference, as distinguished from simple sensory perception. It is prey to many disorders.

2. Fantasy

   Fantasy, or phantasy, is a fabricated series of mental pictures or sequences of events; daydreaming.

   a. Fantasy may express unconscious conflict, gratify otherwise unobtainable wishes, or provide an escape from reality.
   b. It may serve as the springboard for creative activities.
   c. It may lead to a harmful distortion of reality.

3. Phobias

   Phobias are persistent, obsessive fears of specific objects, activities, or situations. Examples include fear of height, closed spaces, open spaces, strangers, animals, dirt, or school. Certain fears, as of harmless bugs and snakes, are extremely common, and not considered pathological, but phobias are typically found in phobic disorders.

4. Obsessions

   Obsessions, also called ruminations, are persistent, recurring ideas or impulses that remain conscious despite their irrationality. Typically found in obsessive-compulsive disorders.

5. Preoccupations

   Preoccupations are excessive concerns with one's own thoughts; engrossment.

6. Delusions

   Delusions are fixed, false beliefs that are not in keeping with the individual's cultural or intellectual level. Found in various types of psychotic disorders—organic mental disorders, schizophrenic disorders, and certain of the affective disorders. They may be—

   a. *Persecutory*, a belief that one is singled out for oppression, attack, or harassment.
   b. *Grandiose*, an exaggerated belief in one's own importance.
   c. *Somatic*, a deluded interpretation of physical symptoms.
   d. *Referential*, a belief that the irrelevant remarks or acts of others refers to oneself.
   e. *Influential*, a belief that one can control or be controlled by another's behavior or thoughts, most commonly observed in paranoid or schizophrenic disorders.
      (1) Ideas of *active influence*, the psychotic belief that one controls others.
      (2) Ideas of *passive influence*, the psychotic belief that one is being controlled by others.
   f. *Nihilistic*, the belief that oneself, the environment, or the world does not exist.
   g. *Self-accusatory*, the belief that one is responsible for harm.
   h. *Other types of delusions* include sin, guilt, impoverishment, illness, and infidelity.

7. Blocking

   Blocking is difficulty in recalling or interpreting a stream of speech or thought because of emotional forces which are usually conscious. Most often found in schizophrenics who, for example, may stop talking, or block, while listening to an imaginary voice or because of conflicting reactions to the message.

8. Magical thinking

   Magical thinking is the imputation of reality to a thought. "Wishing will make it so" is a primitive, prelogical idea believed by small children, encountered in dreams, and found in the thinking of obsessive-compulsive patients.

9. Incoherence

   Incoherence is disorderly, illogical thought, sometimes manifested as garbled speech. Found in schizophrenic disorders, manic disorders, and certain organic mental disorders.

10. Irrelevance

    Irrelevance is thinking that is erroneous or irrelevant to the subject at hand.

11. Circumstantiality
    Circumstantiality is incidental or adventitious thinking. The individual cannot distinguish essentials from nonessentials, although the goal of the thinking is ultimately reached. Commonly found in manic disorder and some organic mental disorders.
12. Tangentiality
    Tangentiality is inability to reach the goal of the thinking.
13. Perseveration
    Perseveration is a persistent, repetitive expression of a single idea in response to various questions. Found in some organic mental disorders and in certain types of catatonia.
14. Condensation
    Condensation is the coalition of several concepts into one.
15. Psychomotor retardation
    Psychomotor retardation is the slowing down of mental and physical activity. Most commonly observed in depressive disorders, but also in some schizophrenic disorders.
16. Psychomotor excitement
    Psychomotor excitement is a mentally and physically hyperactive response to internal or external stimuli. Found in manic disorders and in some catatonic schizophrenic disorders.
17. Flight of ideas
    The *flight of ideas* is skipping from one idea to another in quick succession, without reaching the goal of the thinking. Most commonly observed in the manic disorders.
18. Autism
    Autism, or dereism, is a persistent overindulgence in fantasy. Found in child schizophrenics (pervasive developmental disorders).
19. Misidentification
    Misidentification is the incorrect identification of other people. Found in certain psychotic disorders.
20. Intellectualization
    Intellectualization is the overuse of intellectual concepts and words to avoid feeling or expressing of emotion. Found in adolescents who want to escape their sexual impulses, borderline personalities, obsessive-compulsive patients and some schizophrenics.
21. Clang association
    Clang association is a disturbance in thinking in which the sound of a word, rather than its meaning, sets off a new train of thought. Occurs most often in manic disorders.

G. Disturbances of speech and verbal behavior
   1. Blocking (see "Disturbances of Thinking")
   2. Flight of ideas: (see "Disturbances of Thinking")

3. Logorrhea
Logorrhea, or volubility, is uncontrollable, rapid, excessive talking. Most commonly observed in manic disorders.
4. Pressure of speech
Pressure of speech is rapid, accelerated, voluble speech that is difficult to interrupt. Sometimes found in manic disorders.
5. Neologism
A *neologism* is a coined word or a condensation of several words to express a complex idea. Often known simply as jargon, it is also found in certain schizophrenic disorders.
6. Wordsalad
Wordsalad is an incomprehensible and incoherent mixture of words and phrases. Found in some schizophrenic disorders.
7. Echolalia
Echolalia is the pathological repetition of the phrases or words of another person. Found in some schizophrenic disorders, certain organic mental disorders, and in mental retardation.
8. Echopraxia
Echopraxia is the pathological repetition or imitation of movements the subject is observing. Found in catatonic disorders.
9. Verbigeration
Verbigeration is the meaningless repetition of incoherent words or sentences. Observed in certain psychotic reactions and in certain organic mental disorders.
10. Condensation
Condensation is the contraction of several different ideas into one phrase, forming a collage of thought.

H. Disturbances of motor behavior, or conation
1. Definition
Conation is the basic striving of an individual as expressed in his or her behavior.
2. Psychomotor retardation (see "Disturbances of Thinking")
3. Psychomotor excitement (see "Disturbances of Thinking")
4. Agitation (see "Disturbances of Affect")
5. Echopraxia (see "Disturbances of Verbal Behavior")
6. Catalepsy
Catalepsy is a generalized diminished responsiveness or immobility characterized by trance-like states. Found in organic mental disorders and certain psychogenic disorders.
7. Waxyflexibility
Waxyflexibility, or cerea flexibilitas, is a condition in which a patient passively retains the position into which he or she has been placed. Often present in catatonia.
8. Stereotypy
Stereotypy is the persistent repetition of a motor activity. Sometimes found in schizophrenic disorders.

9. Posturizing

Posturizing is the assumption and maintenance of an unusual posture, often an uncomfortable one. Most commonly observed in catatonics.

10. Mannerisms

Mannerisms are stereotyped movements such as blinking, grimacing, and gesturing. Found in schizophrenic disorders.

11. Negativism

Negativism is opposition, resistance, or refusal to accept reasonable suggestions or advice; a tendency to be in opposition. It may be passive or active. Its most extreme form is found in catatonic schizophrenic disorders.

12. Mutism

Mutism is a form of negativism characterized by refusal to speak, either for conscious or unconscious reasons. Observed in catatonic schizophrenic disorders, profound depressive disorders, and stupors of organic or psychogenic origin.

13. Automatism

Automatism is unconsciously directed automatic, repetitious, and symbolic behavior observed in schizophrenic, convulsive, and dissociative disorders.

I. Disturbances of attention

1. Definition

Attention is the maintenance of focused consciousness to the salient characteristics of the environment.

2. Decreased attention

Decreased attention may result from a lack of interest in or a deliberate shutting out of impinging stimulation.

3. Preoccupation

Preoccupation is concentration on one's own problems which may diminish attention.

4. Fluctuation

Fluctuation of attention is a greater than normal variation, sometimes to the point of inability to attend in spite of the attempt to do so.

5. Blunting of attention

Blunting of attention is extreme inattention, so that even noxious stimulation may not elicit a response.

6. Increased attention

Increased attention, or hyperprosexia, is unusual attention, usually to details of personal significance.

7. Distractibility

Distractibility is a heightened rapid fluctuation of attention, so that every new stimulus, regardless of its significance, is responded to by rapid shifts.

IV. Usefulness of symptomatology
    A. Knowledge of the preceding symptoms is of importance in examining the mental status of the psychiatric patient.
    B. The symptomatology helps to establish a working diagnosis and a treatment program.

References

Freedman, A. M.; Kaplan, H. I.; and Sadock, B. J. *Modern Synopsis of Comprehensive Textbook of Psychiatry,* vol. 2. Baltimore: Williams & Wilkins Company, 1976, chap. 12.

Henderson, D., and Gillespie, R. D. *Textbook of Psychiatry*, 8th ed. London: Oxford University Press, 1956.

Kolb, L. C. *Modern Clinical Psychiatry*, 9th ed. Philadelphia: W. B. Saunders Company, 1977, chap. 6.

Soloman, P., and Patch, V. D. *Handbook of Psychiatry*. Los Altos, Calif.: Lang Medical Publications, 1971, chap. 5.

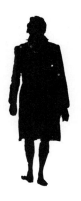

Don't be forecasting evil unless it is what you can guard against. Anxiety is good for nothing if we can't turn it into a defense.

Anxiety

Samuel Meyerick (1783-1848)

I. Introduction

Anxiety plays a key role in psychodynamics and psychopathology. It is also helpful in understanding personality development (see chapter "Psychodynamic Concepts"). It usually plays a major role in normal development as well as in the pathological processes at all ages.

II. Definition

A. *Websters Third New International Dictionary* (1971) defines *anxiety* as "a state of being anxious or of experiencing a strong or dominating blend of uncertainty, agitation, or dread and rooting fear about some contingency; uneasiness."

B. Psychiatrically, *anxiety* can be defined as a diffuse, unpleasant uneasiness, apprehension, or fearfulness stemming from anticipated danger, the source of which is unidentifiable.

III. Character of anxiety

A. Anxiety is really an alerting process, warning the individual of impending danger and stimulating him or her to deal with the threat.

B. It is a highly distressing psychic state, and for this reason one is usually unable to tolerate the symptoms for any sustained period. To deal with it, or manage it, an individual usually enlists one of the coping mechanisms or one of the defense mechanisms.

C. Anxiety is similar to fear.
  1. Both are felt responses to danger and have similar physiologic reactions.
  2. The distinction between anxiety and fear, the fortuitous result of an error in translating the word *angst* from Freud's original work into English, has been overdrawn. Apparently Freud himself did not distinguish appreciably between the two.
  3. Nevertheless, anxiety, in the psychiatric sense, differs from fear. Anxiety is (a) intrapsychic, from within the personality, in origin; (b) a response to an unknown or unrecognized threat; (c) conflictual; and (d) often chronic.

D. Anxiety produces physiological changes during which the body is alerting itself and preparing for vigorous bodily activity (fight or flight).
  1. Certain bodily processes are stimulated and others are inhibited.
    a. The cardiovascular system is stimulated. The heart beats faster and blood pressure is maintained or elevated to force more blood to the muscles. The liver secretes sugar and the adrenal glands produce epinephrine.
    b. The gastrointestinal system is inhibited. Its secretions and peristaltic activity are reduced.

2. These bodily adjustments prepare the organism for activity. The blood that is temporarily removed from the gastrointestinal tract is made available to the muscular system.
3. Biological and psychological defenses are mobilized by anxiety to ensure survival.

IV. Role of anxiety

A. Anxiety occupies a focal position in the dynamics of all human adjustment.
  1. It is a normal response to threat.
  2. It is the driving force for most of our adjustments. For example, anxiety resulting from concern about financial security may: (a) drive one individual to accumulate excessive wealth, (b) stimulate another to plan a realistic investment, insurance, and retirement program, and (c) cause still a third individual to become completely dependent.
  3. The pattern for developing anxiety is inborn and always available. Evidence of this has been noted by child psychiatrists, who have described the underlying *universal* anxieties that are normally associated with the infants anaclitic dependency on the mother.
    a. *Separation anxiety* is the apprehension noted in infants when they are removed from their mothers or mother surrogates. It is most marked from the sixth to the tenth month.
    b. *Stranger anxiety* is the apprehension noted in infants when they are approached by strangers.
    c. *Nocturnal anxiety* is the infant's fear of the dark.
B. The mechanisms for coping with anxiety and the defenses against it form the basis of psychodynamics and psychopathology. These are discussed in the following chapter, "Adaptations to Anxiety."
C. The consistent utilization of certain defenses leads to the development of personality characteristics or character traits (see chapter, "Personality Disorders").

V. Origins of anxiety

A. Otto Rank regarded the trauma of birth as the primary cause of anxiety.
B. The emotional trauma of separations (e.g., anxiety produced by separation from mother or other important supportive nurturing persons in life) is also regarded as the principal origin of anxiety.
C. The response is considered by some to be a learned response.

VI. Components of anxiety

A. Anxiety is present at three different levels.
  1. Neuroendocrine
    Neuroendocrine refers to the chief hormone adrenaline, or epinephrine, secreted by the medulla of the adrenal glands. It

is related to norepinephrine which, in turn, is related to mood disturbance and depression. It accounts for the physiological responses listed below.

2. Psychic

The *psychic* manifestation of anxiety is the sensation of apprehension and the cortical perception of discomfort. It thus includes the appreciation of the physical responses as well as the awareness of the apprehension.

    a. Although the individual consciously perceives and realizes the apprehensiveness, the cause of the anxiety usually escapes awareness.

    b. There are degrees of anxiety (see "Disturbances of Affect" in the previous chapter).

3. Somatic

The *somatic*, or motor-visceral, manifestations of anxiety are the result of the physiological responses of the various bodily systems to the increased secretion of epinephrine.

    a. *Dermatological response.* The skin becomes pale, sweat is secreted, the skin hairs become erect, and there is a shivering of the superficial musculature.

    b. The *cardiovascular response* usually includes tachycardia or palpitations, an increase in systolic blood pressure, and premature contractions. Occasionally, the cardiovascular response is one of decreased activity, with resulting faintness.

    c. *Gastrointestinal response.* The salivary glands are inhibited, with resultant dryness of the mouth. In addition, the individual may experience a foul taste in the mouth, anorexia, nausea, vomiting, cramps, distension, "butterflies in the stomach," diarrhea, or constipation.

    d. The *respiratory response* may include rapid breathing, sighing, or hyperventilation (see "Hyperventilation Syndrome" in the chapter, "Psychosomatic Reactions.")

    e. The *genitourinary response* may include urinary urgency, urinary frequency, dysmenorrhea, dyspareunia, frigidity, impotence, or pelvic pain.

    f. The *vasomotor response* may be sweating or flushing.

    g. The *musculoskeletal response* may be manifested as trembling muscles (often first seen in the lips), dilation of the nostrils, tension headache, constriction in the back of the neck (cervical muscle tension), quavering voice, complaints of arthritis or arthralgia, or various other symptoms in muscles or joints.

    h. The *pupillary response* is dilation (mydriasis).

VII. Responses to anxiety

There is wide variance in individual patterns of response to anxiety.

A. Behavioral

Some individuals evince only behavioral reactions, such as hyper-alertness, irritability, fidgetiness, overdependency, preoccupation, or constriction of activity or concentration

B. Somatic

1. Some have primarily *visceral* reactions in one or more of a number of systems, e.g., the cardiovascular system, the gastrointestinal tract, the genitourinary system, the respiratory system.
2. Others may have symptoms primarily of *muscular tension*, e.g., backache, pain in the joints, or headache due to cervical muscle spasm.
3. Others might have *combinations* of visceral and muscular responses.
4. Why different organ systems are involved in different patients remains incompletely understood.

VIII. Stresses that create anxiety

Theoretically, anxiety can result from all sorts of stimuli (psychosocial stressors) without any awareness on the part of the individual.

A. Anxiety can occur from conflict between

1. The external world and the ego (extrapsychic).
2. The instinctual drives and the censoring forces (intrapsychic).

B. Cultural factors can play an important role in the production of anxiety.

C. Psychosocial stressors are often highly individual. They depend upon the following.

1. The individual's vulnerability.
2. The nature of the stress.
3. The individual's ego resources, including capacity to cope and available defenses.
4. If one's ego functions effectively, one can adapt satisfactorily.

IX. The meaning of anxiety

A. Anxiety is essential to survival. It is emotional pain that serves as a warning or an alert, like physical pain.

B. Anxiety is often a protective symptom. One could view an emotional world without anxiety as very similar to a physical world without friction.

C. During personality development, various adjustive mechanisms evolve to protect the individual from anxiety.

D. Cultural factors—including religion, education, one's value system, and one's degree of sociocultural integration—influence the production of anxiety.

E. If anxiety is severe enough, one is forced to do something about it (move about, take medication, have a drink, see a physician, and so on).

F. Whether anxiety is normal or abnormal depends upon its cause, intensity, and duration.

G. Like physical pain, anxiety can be pathological and is so regarded:
   1. When it is triggered without a known cause or precipitated by a minor event.
   2. When it is unduly persistent and severe.

X. Reducing anxiety

A. Because anxiety is a highly distressing state, individuals usually act to reduce it or be rid of it, by conscious or unconscious mechanisms.
   1. Conscious attempts to control anxiety are often called *coping mechanisms*.
   2. Unconscious ways of dealing with anxiety are called *defenses*.

B. Since much of the symptomatology of the common clinical psychiatric syndromes is based on these various mechanisms, I shall review them briefly in the next chapter before going on to discuss the individual psychiatric disorders.

References

Blum, G. S. *Psychodynamics: The Science of Unconscious Mental Forces*. Belmont, Calif.: Brooks/Cole Publishing Company, 1966, chap. 2.

Eaton, M. T., Jr.; Peterson, M. H.; and Davis, J. A. *Psychiatry*. 3d ed. Flushing, N.Y.: Medical Examination Publishing Company, 1976, chap. 1.

Kolb, L. C. *Modern Clinical Psychiatry*, 9th ed. Philadelphia: W. B. Saunders Company, 1977, chaps. 5, 6.

Solomon, P., and Patch, V. D., eds. *Handbook of Psychiatry*. 2d ed. Los Altos, Calif.: Lang Medical Publications, 1971, chap. 5.

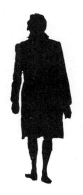

Once more unto the breach, dear friends, once more;
Or close the wall up with our English dead!
In peace there's nothing so becomes a man
As modest stillness and humility:
But when the blast of war blows in our ears,
Then imitate the action of the tiger;
Stiffen the sinews, summon up the blood,
Disguise fair nature with hard-favour'd rage;
Then lend the eye a terrible aspect;
Let it pry through the portage of the head
Like the brass cannon; let the brow o'erwhelm it
As fearfully as doth a galled rock
O'erhang and jutty his confounded base,
Swill'd with the wild and wasteful ocean.
Now set the teeth and stretch the nostril wide,
Hold hard the breath, and bend up every spirit
To his full height! On, on, you noblest English!

Shakespeare: *King Henry V*

Adaptations to Anxiety: Coping and Defense Mechanisms

I. Introduction

A. Individuals usually comport themselves in a fairly predictable, consistent fashion. Although there may be some variation in their behavior, their psychological adaptation is generally in a state of equilibrium. Such a state of emotional poise usually results from their having accumulated a store of problem-solving mechanisms during periods of growth and development. Thus, when they are confronted with the usual stresses of life, called *psychosocial stressors*, they have a variety of effective ways in which to adapt to conflict and frustration.

B. Conscious efforts are regarded as *coping mechanisms. Defense mechanisms* are outside the boundaries of awareness. We are unaware of them as long as they are working well.

C. Most of one's daily frustrations and conflicts can be resolved by conscious and deliberate coping mechanisms. More complex frustrations and conflicts are largely dealt with through unconscious defense mechanisms.

D. We all use defense mechanisms continuously. They are not in themselves pathological unless they are so overused that they distort reality or limit the flexibility of our adaptive behavior. As a matter of fact, defense mechanisms often result in gains: the sublimation of aggressiveness, for example, may result in a successful career in a competitive sport.

II. Definition of defense mechanisms

A. Defense mechanisms are specific, unconscious, intrapsychic adjustments that come into play to resolve emotional conflict and reduce the individual's anxiety.

B. They are also called *mental mechanisms, mental dynamisms, ego defense mechanisms, and adjustive techniques.*

III. Character of defense mechanisms

A. They are automatic, not planned; and economical, not wasted.

B. They have a purpose.
   1. They keep us from becoming anxious or they reduce our anxiety.
   2. They protect the ego.
   3. They maintain repression.

C. They are part of both normal and abnormal adjustments and can be regarded as protective devices.

D. Behavioral theorists would stress the effectiveness of defense mechanisms as avoidance or escape reactions, the learning of which is reinforced by the reduction or termination of aversive stimulation, such as anxiety.

E. Pragmatically, defenses are of two types:
  1. Successful
     Successful defenses are those that eliminate the need for immediate gratification or provide substitute, socially acceptable gratification. Some authorities use the term *sublimation* for successful defenses.
  2. Unsuccessful
     Unsuccessful defenses do not do what is described in 1, and hence do not resolve the conflict and the continuing need for the defense. Thus, there is a repetition of the defense. They also may not reduce the anxiety sufficiently.

IV. **Specific defenses**
  A. Repression
     Repression is the involuntary, automatic banishment of unacceptable ideas, impulses, or feelings into the unconscious (motivated unconscious forgetting).
     1. It is the best known of all the ego defenses and one of the most commonly employed.
     2. It retains the central position in psychodynamic theory that was allotted to it by Freud in relation to ego defenses and symptom formation.
     3. It is sometimes used as a generic term for all defense mechanisms. It is a primary defense against anxiety and as such is considered the cornerstone of psychodynamics. If it is unsuccessful in preventing anxiety, it may then be coupled with other defense mechanisms to permit the emergence of repressed material in disguised form. Two such combinations follow.
        a. *Repression plus displacement,* also termed *focalization,* produces phobic responses that veil the repressed wish. For example, a thirty-six-year-old mother developed the fear that her two-year-old daughter would contract a serious illness. The phobia was a defense against her repressed hostility toward, and rejection of, the girl.
        b. *Repression plus conversion,* also termed *symbolic somatization,* produces an hysterical response. For example, a twenty-year-old soldier developed paralysis of his right hand when firing on the rifle range. His paralysis was a defense against his repressed hostility toward his father; who had abandoned the family.
     4. In psychodynamic theory, conflicts that remain repressed are unchanged in quality and intensity. Because they retain their dynamic drive, they constantly seek expression. This is usually

called *cathexis*. This requires a constant expenditure of emotional energy, *counter-cathexis*, to prevent the conflictual material from appearing in awareness. Often such repressed material re-emerges in other ways: in our dreams, for example, in slips of the tongue, or in other aspects of everyday behavior. Freud referred to these as *the psychopathology of everyday life*.

    5. Not all repressed conflicts cause psychopathology in the individual. Repression is a universally used defense mechanism. For example, we all sometimes forget the name of a well-known person or a frequently called telephone number. Only if abnormal behavior results is repression considered pathological.

B. Suppression

Suppression is the voluntary, intentional relegation of unacceptable ideas or impulses to the foreconscious (volitional exclusion, or conscious forgetting).

    1. Technically, since suppression is a conscious process, it is not considered a true defense mechanism by many authorities.

    2. The conflict can be readily recalled since it remains in the foreconscious.

    3. It is a commonly employed coping mechanism of normal personalities and, thus, is considered a mature defense.

    4. Conscious control requires a strong ego.

    5. Examples of suppression

        a. A person who behaved foolishly under the influence of alcohol the previous evening may consciously try to forget the behavior the following day.

        b. A student who wishes to study for an examination may consciously set aside distracting fantasies.

C. Regression

Regression is the unconscious return to an earlier level of emotional adjustment at which gratification was assured.

    1. The retreat may be partial, total, or symbolic.

    2. Many symptoms of emotional disorder have a regressive aspect, since mature modes of adjustment are replaced by behavior that represents a reversion to an earlier level of adjustment. It is not a desirable adaptation since, in the process, some developmental maturity is lost.

    3. Regression may occur normally, as in the following examples.

        a. It occurs normally in play and sleep.

        b. A toilet-trained, firstborn child may temporarily lose bladder and bowel control in response to the arrival of a second child in the family.

       c. A person promoted to a more responsible position may experience the rearousal of underlying uncertainty, insecurity, and indecision, and hence ask to be returned to the old job.

       d. A person hospitalized for any kind of illness may experience the rearousal of underlying, unmet dependency, and hence make unnecessary requests and demands for attention and care.

   4. Regression may be a symptom of pathology.

       a. Excessive dependence on oral gratification can represent a return to the breast. This is seen, for example, in alcoholics.

       b. It is a primary defense in the production of obsessive-compulsive disorders.

       c. Schizophrenia is profound regression, in the psychological sense. In the more severe forms, regression is seen in many aspects of the individual's personality.

D. Fixation

Fixation is the arrest of maturation at an immature level of psychosexual developmental.

   1. Fixation may occur when there is excessive gratification or excessive frustration at a particular developmental level.

   2. Examples of fixation

       a. An overly dependent attachment to a parent that remains the same over a long period.

       b. Persistence of enuresis into adolescence.

       c. The continued attachment to a nursing bottle beyond infancy.

       d. The infantile behavior sometimes seen in psychosis may be interpreted as fixation or regression.

E. Identification

Identification is the unconscious, wishful adoption, or *internalization,* of the personality characteristics or identity of another individual, generally one possessing attributes that the subject envies or admires.

   1. Normal identification

       a. Identification plays a decisive role in normal personality development, especially the development of the superego (including the conscience), and occurs within the family setting. It requires the continuing presence and emotional support of the parenting ones.

       b. Normally, a boy identifies principally with his father, a girl, with her mother.

       c. Children often emulate other important parent figures, for example, teachers, scout leaders, athletes, or television and movie personalities.

d. A person's adult identification, or *adult individuation,* evolves from the success of identification with all of these important figures.

e. Identification is to be distinguished from *imitation,* which is a conscious mimicking of the behavior of others.

f. *Empathy* is the capacity for participating in, or vicariously experiencing, another's feelings, volitions, or ideas. This ability to feel *with* another is a form of identification found in mature, well-integrated personalities.

g. The *transference* occurring in the therapist-patient relationship in psychotherapy may be based on identification with important figures in one's early life. (See Psychotherapy, in the chapter, "Treatment in Psychiatry.")

2. Identification may be distorted.

a. A person may internalize certain undesirable personality traits of parent or authority figures. This is sometimes called *hostile identification.*

b. *Identification with the aggressor* is the unconscious internalization of the characteristics of a frustrating or feared person.

c. A severely pathological kind of identification is seen in the psychotic person who believes he or she is God or some other important personage.

d. This mechanism operates in shared paranoid disorder, or *folie à deux* (see the chapter, "Paranoid Disorders").

F. Incorporation

Incorporation is a primitive defense mechanism in which the psychic image of another person is wholly or partially assimiliated into an individual's personality. Incorporation is a psychoanalytic term.

1. It is a special type of introjection (see the following).

2. It is the primary mechanism in identification.

3. It is assumed to begin during the oral phase of personality development and to be related to the nursing experience. An example is the infantile fantasy that the mother's breast has been ingested and has become a part of oneself.

G. Introjection

Introjection is the symbolic internalization or assimilation (taking into oneself) of a loved or hated person or external object.

1. This mechanism is the converse of projection (see the following).

2. It is sometimes regarded as a form of identification. It is also closely related to incorporation.

3. It plays a fundamental role in the early development of the ego (it antedates identification).
4. It also plays an important role in the development of the super-ego; that is, the child internalizes parental values and ideals.
5. It operates in the process of *mourning*, sadness appropriate to a loss.
6. It tends to obliterate the distinction between the loved object and the person.
7. Instead of expressing anger or aggression toward others, people sometimes turn these unacceptable tendencies into self-criticism, self-depreciation, and self-accusation. This is also referred to as turning against the self.
8. In depressive disorders, individuals direct unacceptable aggressive and hostile impulses toward themselves—that is, toward the introjected objects or persons within themselves.

H. Projection
Projection is the attributing, to another person or object, the thoughts, feelings, motives, or desires that are really one's own disavowed and unacceptable traits.
   1. Normal projection
      a. Mild forms of projection are normal, everyday activities. We call them alibiing: the "blind" referee, the unfair supervisor, the scapegoat and various prejudices and other types of suspiciousness and hypervigilance to external danger.
      b. In mythology, human qualities are often attributed to non-human things or events. This is also called anthropomorphism. In the novel *Main Street*, by Sinclair Lewis, Carol Kennicott takes a walk in Gopher Prairie shortly after her arrival. Looking up the street, "oozing out from every drab wall, she felt a forbidding spirit which she could never conquer."
      c. Many of us are often critical of our own shortcomings in other people and, as a consequence, tend to hold others responsible for our own difficulties.
   2. Projection as a symptom
      a. To some extent, projection, like rationalization (see the following), is a misinterpretation or distortion of reality, and hence is potentially dangerous.
      b. It is associated with immaturity and vulnerability.
      c. It is a form of displacement and closely associated with denial (see the discussion of denial on page 59).

d. In a pathological sense, this is the mechanism operating in paranoid disorders of all types (paranoia, shared paranoid disorder, paranoid state, paranoid schizophrenia). If the ego becomes disorganized, it leads to
   (1) Delusions or *projected ideation.* The ego loses the capacity to distinguish inner fantasies from external reality.
   (2) Hallucinations, or projections of perception.
   (3) Ideas of reference, also a projection of ideation.

I. Rationalization

Rationalization is the ascribing of acceptable or worthwhile motives to one's own thoughts, feelings, or behavior that really have unrecognized motives. One does something and invents a reason for the action. It can also be thought of as unconscious, retrospective justification.

1. Rationalization, which is an unconscious mechanism, is not to be confused with pretending or lying, both of which are conscious processes because the individual recognizes that the "reasons" for his or her behavior are fictitious.
2. It is a very common defense. Much of our behavior has multiple determinations; that is, several motives are involved. When we "explain" our behavior by the most acceptable of these motives, we are rationalizing.
3. It helps one preserve self-respect and avoid accountability and guilt.
4. It can even be positive in that it enhances self-esteem.
5. A minor element of truth is often involved.
6. Although rationalizing is self-protective, it is also self-deceiving and hence potentially dangerous. As J. B. S. Haldane has written, "let him beware of him in whom reason has become the greatest and most terrible of passions."
7. Examples of rationalization
   a. Punishing someone else, personally or legally, may be a rationalization.
   b. Imbibing extra cocktails may involve rationalization.
   c. The teenager who does not know how to dance, but really wants to, may say that he prefers to stay home.
   d. The "sour grapes" response is a rationalization. In Aesop's fable, *The Fox and the Grapes,* the fox, who was very hungry, strove to obtain some "charming ripe grapes." He failed, then said "let him who will take them!. . ."they are green and sour."

J. Intellectualization

Intellectualization is the overuse of intellectual concepts and words to avoid affective experience or expressions of feelings.

1. It is closely related to rationalization.
2. It is a way of controlling affects and feelings by thinking about them instead of experiencing them.
3. Examples of intellectualization
   a. The adolescent who wants to avoid acknowledging his or her sexual impulses.
   b. Borderline personalities.
   c. Patients suffering from obsessive-compulsive disorders.

K. Compensation

Compensation is a conscious or unconscious attempt to overcome real or fancied inferiorities.

1. Status seems to be an important need in all of us, thus compensatory behavior is universal.
2. Compensation may be—
   a. *Socially acceptable.* For example, the blind person who becomes proficient in music; the paraplegic who becomes successful in politics.
   b. *Socially unacceptable.* For example, the physically handicapped person who becomes a bully or a boor; the physically small person who becomes aggressive and domineering ("the small man syndrome" or "the banty rooster syndrome").
3. Compensation may also be—
   a. *Direct*, that is, an attempt to achieve in an area in which one has failed.
   b. *Indirect*, that is, an attempt to achieve in a different field than the field in which one has failed.
4. *Overcompensation* is an exaggerated attempt to overcome inferiorities.
5. William Wordsworth (1770–1850) in *Character of the Happy Warrior,* describes compensation:
   "who, doomed to go in company with
   pain
   and Fear, and Bloodshed, miserable
   train!
   Turns his necessity to glorious gain!"

L. Reaction formation

Reaction formation is the direction of overt behavior or attitudes in precisely the opposite direction of the individual's underlying, unacceptable conscious or unconscious impulses.

1. It is a two-step defense.
   a. An unacceptable desire is repressed.
   b. The repression is followed by the conscious expression of its antithesis.
2. The conscious intent of reaction formation is often altruistic.
3. The use of this adaptive pattern often leads to the production of lasting changes in an individual's behavior. For example:
   a. Uriah Heep, the hypocritical clerk in Charles Dickens' *David Copperfield,* insists that he is a very "humble" person, but his underlying nature is detestable, sly, and conniving.
   b. "Don Juan's" may be masking underlying doubts about their masculinity.
   c. Excessive politeness or courtesy may disguise underlying hostility.
   d. Overt oversolicitousness and overprotectiveness toward a child may hide a parent's hostile and rejecting feelings.
   e. Submissiveness, excessive amiability, or excessive concern may be reaction formations against underlying hostility or aggressiveness.
   f. Compulsive meticulousness may cover up strong impulses to soil.
M. Sublimation
   Sublimation is the diversion of unacceptable, instinctual drives into socially sanctioned channels.
   1. This is socialization of emotion.
   2. It is a term often reserved for successful defense mechanisms because, while the underlying impulse is gratified and the goal is retained, they are redirected from socially unacceptable to socially acceptable paths.
   3. Unlike other defenses, there is no counter cathexis. The emotional energy from an unacceptable impulse is transferred to a new goal-directed activity that is decided upon by the ego and approved by the super-ego.
   4. Since sublimation offers some gratification of the underlying instinctual drive, it is usually considered healthy and often regarded as the most desirable of the mental mechanisms.
   5. Examples of sublimation
      a. Sports and games may be sublimations of hostile and aggressive impulses.
      b. Various types of creative activity may be sublimations of sexual drives.
      c. Vocational choices may be sublimations of underlying unacceptable impulses.

N. Denial

Denial is the unconscious disavowal of a thought, feeling, wish, need, or reality that is consciously unacceptable. One behaves as if the problem does not exist. Denial is to be distinguished from *lying,* which is a conscious process.

1. Dynamically, denial is the simplest form of ego defense, closely related to rationalization.
2. It is a very primitive defense mechanism, much used by young children. The shutting of the infant's eyes, to avoid seeing a threatening situation, is the prototype of this defense.
3. Denial is also sometimes used to defend oneself against catastrophe.
4. It is also much used by deteriorated psychotics, who may replace the rejected reality with a more satisfying fantasy.
5. Examples of denial
   a. The small child who disclaims pain when a finger has been smashed in the door.
   b. The deaf individual who refuses to admit a hearing loss.
   c. The alcoholic who refuses to admit that he or she cannot handle liquor.
   d. The dissatisfied employee who believes that a change in jobs will solve all of his or her vocational problems.

O. Substitution

Substitution is an unconscious replacement of a highly valued but unattainable or unacceptable emotional goal or object by one that is attainable or acceptable.

1. It is comparable to displacement.
2. To be satisfactory, the substitutive activity must have certain similarities to the original forbidden one. For example, murderous or intensely hostile impulses may be replaced by some impersonal destructive act, such as striking a punching bag or shooting a target rifle.

P. Restitution

Restitution is the supplanting of a highly valued object that has been lost through rejection by, or death or departure of, another object.

1. It is really a special form of substitution.
2. An example is the second marriage of a widowed person.

Q. Displacement

Displacement is the redirection of an emotion from the original object to a more acceptable substitute.

1. It is closely allied to symbolization (see symbolization on page 61).

2. It is normal, as when hostile feelings are transferred from an employer to some member of the family or some other object or when various feelings are displaced onto political figures or certain minority groups.
3. Feelings of hostility to parents are also often transferred to parent surrogates or other authority figures.
4. It also occurs in the transference-countertransference relationship in psychiatric treatment.
5. It is found in phobic disorders, where there is transference of anxiety from an unconscious conflict to an external focus.
6. It is frequently found in obsessive-compulsive disorders. For example, handwashing may result from feelings of moral uncleanness. These feelings are displaced onto dirt, which must be continually cleansed away.

R. Isolation

Isolation is the separation of an unacceptable impulse, act, or idea from its memory origin, thereby removing the emotional charge associated with the original memory.
1. The idea is set apart from its attached original affect, by counter-cathexis.
2. Isolation differs from repression proper, in which the idea as well as the feeling tone is kept out of awareness.
3. Although the individual consciously retains, or can recall, the painful memory of a traumatic incident, the feeling that originally accompanied it has become detached.
4. This mechanism is commonly seen in obsessive-compulsive disorder. Characteristically, the obsessive-compulsive person remains emotionally aloof from loaded situations. For example,
   a. An obsessed person feels he or she might hurt or kill someone but not have the accompanying hostile or aggressive feelings.
   b. It is the basis of many compulsive rituals.
5. It is found in the compartmentalization of two ideas, that are antithetical as, for example, in the devoutly religious person who shows racial prejudice.

S. Undoing

Undoing is a primitive defense mechanism in which some unacceptable past behavior is symbolically acted out in reverse, usually repetitiously. It is also called *symbolic atonement*.
1. It is nullification by counteraction.
2. It is treating an experience as if it had never occurred.
3. It is closely related to reaction formation (magical expiation).
4. Examples of undoing
   a. An executive who has recommended that an employee not be promoted later makes complimentary remarks to the person.

b. A person with an obsessive-compulsive disorder may undo the hostility shown at the beginning of an interview by being ingratiating at the end of the interview.

c. Handwashing may represent expiation for antisocial or asocial activities. Repetition compulsion represents an attempt to reenact earlier unacceptable emotional experiences in order to be freed from their original unconscious meaning.

T. Dissociation

Dissociation is the unconscious detachment of certain behavior from the normal or usual conscious behavior patterns of an individual, which then function alone (compartmentalization). It is seen normally—

1. In the executive who keeps his or her business from interfering with family life.
2. In sleepwalking, or somnambulism, sleeptalking, and automatic behavior such as automatic handwriting.
3. In the dissociative disorders, such as psychogenic amnesia, psychogenic fugue, and depersonalization disorder.
4. In multiple personalities, for example, in *Dr. Jekyll and Mr. Hyde* or *The Three Faces of Eve*. Generally, the primary character is proper and moral, whereas the secondary personality is hedonistic and impulse-ridden.
5. In schizophrenia, where there is a splitting of affect from mental content.

U. Symbolization

Symbolization is the unconscious mechanism by which a neutral idea or object is used to represent another idea or object that has a forbidden aspect.

1. There is a displacement of emotion from the object to the symbol.
2. Symbolization is based on similarity and association. The symbols protect the individual from the anxiety attached to the original idea or object.
3. Symbolization is the language of the unconscious.
4. Examples of symbolization
   a. Dreams are the most common examples of symbolization. In dreams, for example,
      (1) Elongated or projecting objects are often phallic symbols.
      (2) Openings or shrubbery may represent female genitalia.
      (3) A ship, ocean, or mothering figure may represent the mother.
   b. Affectations of speech, dress, or gait may be symbolizations.
   c. Certain psychotic symptoms such as hallucinations, muteness, posturizing, and sterotopy may have symbolic meaning.

V. Idealization

Idealization is the over-estimation of admired qualities of another person or desired object. It is normally seen in—
1. Young persons who exaggerate the intelligence and attractiveness of their friends or lovers.
2. Precinct workers who overevaluate the assets and underestimate the limitations of a political candidate.

W. Fantasy

Fantasy is a fabricated series of mental pictures or sequence of events; daydreaming.
1. Fantasy may provide the basis for creative activities.
2. Daydreams can express unconscious conflict, gratify otherwise unattainable wishes, provide an escape from reality.
3. A disproportionate preoccupation with fantasy may lead to harmful distortion of reality.

V. Special defense mechanisms

Because of the current interest in borderline and narcissistic personalities (see the chapter, "Personality Disorders"), two additional defense mechanisms are of importance. They are primitive or psychotic defenses that support denial much in the way that displacement, introjection, sublimation, and the other defenses support repression. These defenses are

A. Splitting

Splitting is the inability to unite and integrate the hating and loving aspects of both one's self-image and one's image of another person. The loving, fantasied, relationships and the hating ones are internally "split." When the individual develops positive fantasies, the negative feelings are dissociated or "split off"; when the person is frustrated, the negative fantasies are elaborated.

B. Projective identification

Projective identification is the association of uncomfortable aspects of one's own personality with their projection onto another person, resulting in identification with the other person.

C. For further discussion of these concepts see E. R. Shapiro, cited in the References that follow this chapter.

VI. Summary

The foregoing are not all of the defenses against anxiety that have been described by various authorities, but they do include the principal mechanisms seen in the day-to-day adjustments of normal persons as well as in the major psychiatric syndromes.

References

Blum, G. S. *Psychodynamics: The Science of Unconscious Mental Forces.* Belmont, Calif.: Brooks/Cole Publishing Company, 1966.

Eaton, M. T., Jr.; Peterson, M. H.; and Davis, J. A. *Psychiatry.* 3d ed. Flushing, N.Y.: Medical Examination Publishing Company, 1976, chap. 1.

Freedman, A. M.; Kaplan, H. I., and Sadock, B. J. *Modern Synopsis of Comprehensive Textbook of Psychiatry.* Baltimore: Williams & Wilkins Company, 1976, pp. 255–56.

Freud, A. *The Ego and the Mechanisms of Defense.* New York: International University Press, 1953.

Kolb, L. C. *Modern Clinical Psychiatry.* 9th ed. Philadelphia: W. B. Saunders Company, 1977, chap. 5.

Shapiro, E. R. "The Psychodynamics and Developmental Psychology of a Borderline Patient: A Review of the Literature." *American Journal of Psychiatry.* November, 1978, 135.

Solomon, P., and Patch V. D., eds. *Handbook of Psychiatry.* 2d ed. Los Altos, Calif.: Lang Medical Publications, 1971, chap. 31.

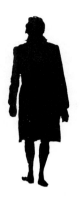

Anxiety Disorders

My apprehensions come in crowds;
I dread the rustling of the grass;
The very shadows of the clouds
Have power to shake me
   as they pass;
I question things and do not find
One that will answer to my mind;
And all the world appears unkind.

William Wordsworth: *The Affliction
of Margaret (1804)*

I. Definition
A. *Anxiety disorders* were formerly classified as neuroses or neurotic disorders.
B. In this group of disorders, some form of anxiety is either:
  1. The most prominent disturbance in the clinical picture, as in panic disorder and generalized anxiety disorder; or
  2. Experienced because the individual tries to resist succumbing to his other symptoms, as in avoidance of a dreaded object or situation (in a phobic disorder) and obsessions or compulsions (in an obsessive compulsive disorder).

II. Introduction
A. Anxiety disorders represent an individual's unsuccessful compromise efforts to deal with underlying primitive needs.
B. Since anxiety is the central force in these disorders, they are characterized chiefly by the symptomatic expression of anxiety or the defenses by which the ego tries to control the anxiety.
C. Symptoms of anxiety include:
  1. Panic
  2. Apprehensive anticipation
  3. Motor tension
  4. Avoidance behavior
  5. Vigilance behavior

III. Character of anxiety disorders
A. Repression is incomplete in the anxiety disorders.
B. The relationships between the symptoms and underlying conflicts are usually unrecognized by the individual.
C. The choice of defenses is in part a product of the individual's character structure, and thus, according to psychoanalytic theory, is determined by the developmental stage in which fixation occurred or from which the person's most prominent character traits were derived.
D. In some of these disorders, the "neurotic" compromise is never completely satisfactory because the defenses employed produce symptoms (e.g., phobias, obsessions, or compulsions) that are distressful and from which the individual seeks relief.

IV. Etiology
A. Biologic and genetic factors are not thought to be of major significance in anxiety disorders.
B. Social factors are felt by many to play some role. Cultural forces and family interactions seem to play a part in many of these disorders. Some psychiatrists feel that the family unit, rather than the individual, is the proper focus of treatment.

C. Psychogenic factors, both antecedent and concurrent, are regarded by most authorities as the basic etiological factors.
1. Antecedent factors

Antecedent factors operating during the early developmental years seem to be the most significant. These include parental attitudes toward the child and the child's feelings about whether or not he or she was accepted and loved.
   a. The infant's long period of dependency on the mother seems to be a crucial factor.
   b. Disturbances of the child-parent relationship in the earliest years seem particularly significant; for example, a parent who is harsh, overprotective, or inconsistent.
   c. Behavior such as sleepwalking, enuresis, and nailbiting often characterize the childhood of these individuals.
   d. Thus, the therapist tries to connect the current symptomatology with some unresolved childhood conflict.
2. Concurrent factors

Concurrent factors, i.e., precipitating or immediate causes that trigger or initiate the disorders, are often evident in the development of the symptoms, which are frequently hostile, sexual, or dependent feelings.
   a. Reality may be a precipitant rather then a cause.
   b. The dehumanizing aspects of modern-day society may be a psychological threat.
3. Therapists usually regard the etiology as a constellation of factors rather than a single cause. A more detailed outline of etiology is given in the sections of this chapter describing the various types of anxiety disorders, but there are, largely, two approaches to the problem.
   a. Dynamic

   The *dynamic* point of view is largely psychoanalytic in orientation. Anxiety is regarded as the central force in the production of these disorders, and various symptoms are thought to result from the manner in which the ego deals with anxiety.
   b. Physiologic

   The *physiologic* point of view is that these disorders are conditioned responses resulting from stressful stimuli with which the individual is unable to cope.

V. Prevalence

A. It is estimated that 2 to 4 percent of the general population has at some time had a disorder described as either an "anxiety state" or a "phobia." In *The Diagnostic and Statistical Manual of Mental*

Disorders, 3d ed. (*DSM*-III), it is estimated that approximately 10 percent of patients in cardiology practice are suffering from an anxiety disorder.

    B. Most anxiety disorders occur during early adult life (from late adolescence to the middle thirties), the period when most people are confronted with the greatest responsibilities and hence have the greatest need for adjustment.

VI. Classification

    A. The category of neuroses is not used as a basis for classification in *DSM*-III. The disorders that formerly were classified as neuroses included in *DSM*-II are now included in anxiety disorders, somatoform disorders, dissociative disorders, affective disorders, and psychosexual disorders.

    B. The anxiety disorders include the following. (Corresponding terms from the *DSM*-II are enclosed in brackets.)

        1. Phobic disorders [phobic neuroses]

            a. Agoraphobia

                (1) Agoraphobia with panic attacks

                (2) Agoraphobia without panic attacks

            b. Social phobia

            c. Simple phobia

        2. Anxiety states [anxiety neuroses]

            a. Panic disorder

            b. Obsessive compulsive disorder [obsessive compulsive neuroses]

            c. Generalized anxiety disorder

            d. Post traumatic stress disorder

    C. The remainder of this chapter is devoted to the anxiety disorders. The somatoform disorders and the dissociative disorders are the subjects of the following two chapters. Depressive disorders are discussed in the chapter on affective disorders.

VII. Phobic disorders [phobic neuroses]

    A. Definition

        1. The essential feature of *phobic disorders* is persistent avoidance behavior secondary to irrational fears of a specific object, activity, or situation.

        2. Synonyms are *phobic neurosis, phobic reaction, phobia.*

        3. The word *phobia* is derived from the Greek Phobos, a god who could provoke fear and panic.

    B. History

        1. Shakespeare described phobic behavior in *The Merchant of Venice:*

        "Some men there are love not a gaping pig:

        Some, that are mad if they behold a cat . . ."

2. In 1872, Westphal published his classic monograph *Agoraphobia* (*Die agoraphobia*).
3. In 1909, Freud described the case of "Little Hans," a five-year-old who developed a phobia.

C. Prevalence
1. About 2 to 3 percent of the cases in psychiatric practice in the United States and England. About half these patients, mostly women, have agoraphobia (see agoraphobia, p. 69).
2. Young children (around the age of three or four) normally have occasional irrational fears of animals or common objects.

D. Symptoms
1. Aside from the phobia itself, the symptoms are ways of avoiding the feared object, activity, or situation. These obviously restrict the individual's freedom of action. The individual has focalized the anxiety and, as long as he or she can avoid the focalized object, activity, or situation, remains relatively comfortable and free of anxiety.
2. The type of fear is in part culturally determined and, as in some conversion disorders, there is a secondary gain factor. For example, fear of airplanes may develop in a person whose job requires air travel.
3. If confronted with the feared object, activity, or situation, the individual develops anxiety that varies in degree from mild uneasiness to panic.
4. The individual recognizes the unreasonableness of the phobia but is unable to control the behavior or explain the fear.
5. There are numerous types of phobias, since they can develop about almost anything.

E. Clinical types
1. Agoraphobia
   a. Definition
      In *DSM*-III *agoraphobia* is defined as a phobic disorder in which the predominant disturbance is an irrational fear of leaving the familiar setting of the home. It is almost always preceded by a phase during which there are recurrent attacks of panic. The individual develops an anticipatory fear of helplessness when having a panic attack and is, therefore, reluctant or refuses to be alone, travel or walk alone, or to be alone in unfamiliar situations such as crowds, closed or open spaces, crowded stores, bridges, tunnels, or churches. These fears are pervasive and dominate the individual's life, so that a large number of situations are entered into only reluctantly or are avoided (thus, there is constriction of normal activities). In the severe form of the disorder, the individual is "housebound." (Thus, there is marked fear of being alone or being in public places.)

b. Subtypes

In the *DSM*-III agoraphobia is classified as occuring with panic attacks and without panic attacks. (Thus, there is marked fear of being alone or being in public places.)

c. Associated features

(1) Patients commonly insist that a family member or a friend accompany them whenever they leave home ("phobic partner").

(2) Agoraphobia is almost always accompanied by nonphobic symptoms such as anxiety, panic, or feelings of depersonalization.

d. Prevalence

One study indicates that about 5 percent of the population has at some time suffered from agoraphobia.

e. Predisposing factor

Phobic disorder and separation anxiety disorder in childhood.

f. Case example

Mrs. A. W., the forty-eight-year-old wife of a small-town physician, sought psychiatric treatment because she had a fear of being in church. Actually, as she unfolded her story, she really feared leaving the home and, before she developed the fear of going to church, had become uneasy while shopping and driving the children to school. It became evident, during exploratory interviews, that the onset of this agoraphobic behavior was related to her husband's heart attack two years earlier. Since he was several years her senior, she was fearful that he might have a second heart attack that would prove fatal.

As she became aware of the relationship of her symptom to her concern about her husband's health, she was able to respond to a combined approach of psychotropic medication and a program of gradual desensitization. She began by forcing herself to attend a church of her own denomination in a nearby town and then, by degrees, finally forced herself to attend her own church and sit in the front row.

2. Social phobia

a. Definition

Social phobia is a persistent, irrational fear of, and compelling desire to avoid, a situation in which the individual is exposed to possible scrutiny by others and fears that he or she may act in a way that will be humiliating or embarrassing (*DSM*-III). (Fear of situations with potential for public embarrassment.)

b. Prevalence

This disorder is apparently rare.

c. Case example

A twenty-four-year-old single man consulted a psychiatrist because of his fear of speaking before groups of people, particularly in classrooms. He reported that the first episode occurred in the sixth grade, when he was called on to recite in front of his class and that his fearfulness became more evident in high school and worsened during his college days, when he was in smaller classes where more personal participation was demanded. Whenever he had to speak to a group of people, he became shy, nervous, and short of breath.

On examination, he appeared cooperative, pleasant, but unable to look at himself in a psychological way. He did not exhibit any unusual behavior or thinking pattern throughout the interviews and, although somewhat anxious and uneasy to begin with, relaxed later.

Psychological testing revealed that he had superior intelligence and good ego-strengths, but he seemed to view the world about him as a somewhat threatening and conflictual place in which to live. This seemed particularly true of his relationships with men, whom he regarded as competitors. Since his symptoms were not severe and he had good ego-strengths, he was urged to return to school, enroll in a course that required classroom participation, and forcibly confront himself with the situation that might make him fearful.

3. Simple phobia
   a. Definition
      Persistent, irrational fear of, and compelling desire to avoid an object or a situation other than being alone or in public places away from home or of humiliation or embarrassment (*DSM*-III).
   b. Types
      The most common simple phobias involve animals, particularly reptiles, insects, and rodents. Others are *claustrophobia* and *acrophobia* (fear of heights).
F. Psychopathology of phobic disorders
   1. Essentially, in phobic disorders, an individual experiences severe, diffuse anxiety that is only incompletely resolved by repression. Thus there is displacement of the anxiety to an external focus, (focalizing or binding anxiety) which the individual then tries to avoid.
   2. The choice of phobia is sometimes thought to be fortuitous, but it is more commonly thought to be a symbolic representation of the underlying impulse or desire.
      a. The mother who fears she may harm her youngster has an unconscious desire to hurt the child; the person who fears dirt may have underlying desires to soil or to be dirty.

b. Some phobias represent the fear of punishment for the underlying unacceptable desire. For example, a person who is tempted to harm himself or herself because of guilt over hostility to a spouse may develop a fear of knives.
3. A phobic partner, or "obligatory companion," who protects the phobic patient is sometimes dynamically involved in this disorder. Such a partner is viewed as a symbolic parent who helps to satisfy the phobic person's dependency. Many times there seems to be an element of secondary gain for the partner as well.
4. Sometimes the patient develops counterphobic behavior, repeatedly and compulsively confronting himself or herself with the source of anxiety in an attempt to remain in control.
5. From the above, it is evident that the phobic patient uses the following ego defenses: repression, displacement, symbolization, and avoidance (see the chapter, "Adaptations to Anxiety").

G. Course and prognosis
1. Many phobias are chronic; however, if the conflict is close to consciousness and dealt with promptly, the prognosis is good.
2. If the conflict is deep and the phobic reactions are highly disguised or highly symbolic, the prognosis is much more serious.
3. The presence of compulsive symptoms makes the prognosis less hopeful (in some cases, there is little or no difference between this reaction and obsessive-compulsive disorder).
4. In some cases, the phobias tend to spread. This usually occurs when displacement fails to relieve the anxiety and further restricts the individual's behavior.

H. Treatment
1. *Supportive psychotherapy,* including reassurance, suggestion, and emotional support, is often enough to relieve mild phobic responses.
2. Desensitization, deconditioning, or other forms of *behaviorial therapy* have been advocated by some. In these treatments, direct attacks are made on the phobic behavior rather than on the underlying unconscious conflicts.
3. *Insight psychotherapy* is, however, usually necessary in the more serious cases.
4. A combination of a direct attack on the phobia, plus subsequent insight therapy, is sometimes the most practical. This is especially true when the phobia is extremely disruptive of the individual's life.
5. *Group therapy* has been helpful, especially when used in conjunction with deconditioning.
6. *Medications,* including anti-anxiety agents, are helpful in reducing associated anxiety.

VIII. Panic disorders

A. Definition

The essential feature of *panic disorders* is recurrent panic (anxiety) attacks and nervousness. In general, the symptoms are characteristic of widespread, sudden autonomic discharge. The attacks are characterized by a sudden onset of intense apprehension, fearfulness, or terror, often associated with feelings of impending doom (*DSM*-III).

B. Course

The course is recurrent and episodic. The individual is never certain when an attack will occur.

C. Prevalence

The disorder is apparently common.

D. Predisposing factor

Separation anxiety, or anxiety disorder in childhood.

E. Symptoms

In general the symptoms are similar to those of fear, yet there is no employment of defense mechanisms to manage or control the episodes. The most common symptoms experienced are dyspnea; palpitations, chest pains, or discomfort; choking or smothering sensations, dizziness, vertigo, or unsteady feelings; feelings of unreality (depersonalization and derealization); paresthesias; hot and cold flashes; sweating; faintness; trembling or shaking; and fear of dying, going crazy, or doing something uncontrolled during the attack. The attacks usually last minutes or, more rarely, hours (*DSM*-III).

F. Differential diagnoses

Disorders which can produce panic symptoms must be ruled out. (e.g., mitral valve prolapse, hypoglycemia, pheochromocytoma, hyperthyroidism).

G. Psychopathology

1. Anxiety results when some conflict is aroused or rearoused either by a weakening of the repressive forces or by strengthening (or reinforcement) of the underlying drive or wish.
2. Thus, repressed conflicts press for reemergence.
3. The symptoms are nonspecific and do not offer any clues to the underlying etiology. However, the precipitating circumstances and the setting in which attacks occur, especially the first attack, usually give some clues to the underlying cause.

H. Course and prognosis

1. Usually occurs as attacks; between attacks the individual may be comfortable, although more commonly he or she is somewhat tense.
2. If the conflict is not resolved, the individual may utilize one or more of the defense mechanisms and thus develop the picture of one of the other clinical reaction types.

3. Ordinarily, the prognosis is for recurrent espisodes.
4. Some cases become chronic.
5. A panic attack may be the precursor of other mental disorders, such as schizophrenia, major depressive disorder, or somatization disorder.

I. Treatment
1. Short-term supportive psychotherapy
This is usually indicated and includes—
   a. Reassurance and support (not only verbal but attitudinal as well).
   b. Clarification and education, including pointing out various dynamic and stress factors and supporting various positions and recommendations about changes.
   c. Environmental modification, including changing the environment in some way, modifying whatever stresses may be present, and family therapy.

2. Insight psychotherapy
Although most psychotherapy is aimed at giving some insight, certain cases of this disorder may require long-term interpretative, psychoanalytically oriented, psychotherapy.

3. Medications
Reliance is chiefly on the benzodiazipines (Chlordiazepoxide, Diazepam, Oxpam, Lorezepam, and so forth). Neuroleptic agents such as Chlorpromazine or Thioridazine are sometimes prescribed. Antidepressant medications such as the tricyclics may be added if depressive symptoms occur.

4. Deconditioning
Since much anxiety is a conditioned response, deconditioning has been tried with some success (see behavioral therapy in the chapter, "Treatment in Psychiatry").

J. Case example

Mrs. J., a thirty-year-old housewife, sought psychiatric treatment because of the following symptoms: irritability, anxiousness, lower abdominal pain, numbness and tingling of her extremities, and fearfulness about her health. Although she had been a "nervous" person most of her life, her presenting symptoms had begun three months earlier and occurred in "attacks."

During a series of interviews, it was learned that the onset of her symptoms occurred the day her sister unexpectedly removed a niece the patient had been caring for in her home while the mother was hospitalized for delivery of a baby. Two factors in her past history were of dynamic significance: (1) she had been the oldest girl in a large family and cared for the other siblings, especially when her mother was in the hospital having babies; and (2) sterility—she had been unable to conceive during ten years of marriage.

Thus, recurrent anxiety attacks were precipitated in a woman desirous of having a family, who in the past had to "give up" children when the mother returned, and who again had been forced to "give up" a child.

From a dynamic viewpoint, the symptoms were manifestations of the patient's conflict between her desire for children and her inability to conceive. The fact that she had to "give up" a child three months earlier reactivated the conflict and precipitated the symptoms.

In this case, the presenting symptoms were both somatic and psychic, were typical of anxiety, and came in attacks. The conflict was relatively superficial.

IX. Generalized anxiety disorder

A. Definition

The essential feature of generalized anxiety disorder is chronic (at least 6 months), generalized, and persistent anxiety without the specific symptoms that characterize phobic disorders, panic disorder, or obsessive compulsive disorder. The diagnosis is not made when the onset of the disturbance is clearly associated with a psychosocial stressor and when it is assumed that the disturbance will remit if and when the stressor ceases (*DSM*-III). (Persistent and generalized anxiety without panic attacks.)

B. Subtypes

Individuals who have a disturbance of less than six months' duration and those with morbid fear of disease are classified in *DSM*-III as having *atypical anxiety disorder*.

C. Symptoms or clinical features

In general, the symptoms are manifestations of chronic autonomic hyperactivity. They may be of the following categories:

1. Motor tension

Related to increased muscle tone, as shakiness, jitteriness, jumpiness, trembling, tenseness, inability to relax, restlessness, or easy to startle.

2. Autonomic hyperactivity

Different manifestations of sympathetic or parasympathetic activity, as sweating, pounding heart, dry mouth, lightheadedness, tingling feelings in the hands or feet, frequent urination, diarrhea.

3. Apprehensive expectation

Anxiety, worry, fear, rumination, and anticipation of misfortune to self or others

4. Vigilance and scanning

Hyperattentiveness resulting in distractibility, difficulty in concentrating, insomnia, feeling "on edge," irritability, impatience.

D. Course

The long-term course is unknown.

E. Psychopathology

See earlier section, under Panic disorders. By definition in the new *DSM*-III, generalized anxiety disorder is *not* associated with psychosocial stressors.

F. Treatment

See Treatment, under Panic attack.

X. **Obsessive-compulsive disorder** [obsessive compulsive neurosis]

A. Definition

The essential features of obsessive-compulsive disorder are recurrent obsessions, compulsions, or both. The *obsessions* are defined as recurrent and persistent ideas, thoughts, images, or impulses that are ego-dystonic; that is, they are not experienced as voluntarily produced, but rather as ideas that invade the consciousness and are experienced as senseless or repugnant. Attempts are made to ignore or suppress them. *Compulsions* are repetitive and seemingly purposeful behaviors that are performed according to certain rules or in a stereotyped fashion. The behavior is not an end in itself, but is designed to produce or prevent some future event or situation. However, either the activity is not connected in a realistic way with what it is designed to produce or prevent, or may be clearly excessive. The act is performed with a sense of subjective compulsion coupled with a desire to resist the compulsion (at least initially). The individual generally recognizes the senselessness of the behavior (this may not be true for young children) and does not derive pleasure from carrying out the activity, although it provides a release of tension.

B. Prevalence

1. Fleeting obsessions or compulsions are more or less universal.
2. Obsessive-compulsive traits are not uncommon in children and adolescents.
3. In several countries, approximately 2 percent of all psychiatric outpatients carry this diagnosis.
4. The incidence may be somewhat higher because people with this disorder often conceal their symptoms and avoid consulting a physician about them.
5. It is said that a large number of obsessive-compulsive people remain unmarried.
6. Some studies indicate that the reaction is more common among people in the upper socioeconomic class and those of high I. Q.
7. Gender is apparently not a factor.

C. Symptoms

1. The symptoms may take many forms. Doubt and vacillation are prominent.

2. Obsessions

These recurring ideas or impulses can be about anything, but the most common themes are violence, contamination, and doubt. Other themes are sexuality, obscenities, and religion or religious subjects (scrupulosity).

3. Compulsions

These are recurrent, compelling acts that develop in the attempt to relieve obsessions or fears. They are of two types: (1) reactions to or attempts to control the underlying obsession, and (2) direct expressions of the underlying obsessive urges. The second type is rare, and similar to counterphobic measures in phobic patients.

   a. Among common compulsions are counting, checking, and touching.
   b. Other common compulsions include (1) contamination, for example, handwashing rituals that develop as a means of relieving fears of, or obsessions about, dirt or germs, and (2) self-mutilation, for example, self-inflicted excoriations as a compulsive punishment for guilt about masturbation.

4. As can be seen from the foregoing, the obsessions are mainly asocial in nature and the compulsions are mainly "caricatures of morality." In fully developed cases, there is a 50–50 ratio between the obsessions and compulsions. Such a state of dynamic equilibrium explains the underlying indecision, uncertainty, and ambivalence of these patients.

5. Sometimes the symptoms are less specific, being manifested as a compulsive and ritualistic quality that pervades all of the individual's behavior. Thus, some individuals perform certain rituals on arising in the morning, dress according to a certain pattern, or perform daily tasks and duties in a fixed and exact sequence.

6. Sometimes the compelling idea may be neutral or indifferent, and the term *obsessive-ruminative state* is then used. The central rumination is often of a religious or philosophical nature. The matter is repeatedly meditated upon, consideration is given to the pros, cons, and imponderables, but no resolution of the matter is achieved.

7. The patient is often embarrassed about the compulsions and rituals, and may go to great lengths to disguise them from others. If they become more severe or chronic, the person's ability to hide the acts becomes progressively less successful.

8. Depression and anxiety symptoms are common.

D. Psychopathology

Obsessive compulsive disorder is dynamically much more complicated than any of the other anxiety disorders.

1. Repression, for some reason, is unsuccessful or only incompletely successful, and the individual makes use of other defenses to reinforce the repression. These subsequent defenses are isolation, reaction formation, undoing, and displacement (see the chapter, "Adaptations to Anxiety").
2. Ambivalence
   Ambivalence, the coexistence of two opposing feelings toward the same individual or object, is very prominent in obsessive-compulsive patients. The feelings are usually love and hate. Ambivalence is also evident in undoing.
3. Premorbid personality
   The premorbid personality typically has obsessional characteristics. That is, he or she is rigid, restricted, orderly, meticulous, cautious, deliberate, conscientious, and dependable. The person who possesses such compulsive qualities is also referred to as an *anancastic personality,* or *anal character* (an individual who needs to feel in control of himself or herself and of the environment). The presence of these traits does not constitute abnormality. Most of the people who have obsessive-compulsive traits do not become obsessive-compulsive patients.
   a. According to psychoanalytic theorists, such anal qualities develop in the infant during the period of toilet training (the anal phase of infantile sexuality). The development of obsessive-compulsive disorder represents fixation at, or regression to, this anal phase of development—a period when the superego is harsh, demanding, and punitive.
   b. According to learning theorists, obsessions are conditioned responses to anxiety, and compulsions are behavioral patterns that reduce the anxiety.
4. The function of the compulsive act is to allay (relieve) and bind (tie down or focalize) anxiety.
5. The acts are symbolic.
E. Course and prognosis
1. The onset of obsessive-compulsive disorder may occur at any period of life, but commonly begins in adolescence. This is probably because this is a period when there is increased sexual awareness, conflict about dependency and independency, and so forth.
2. Obsessive-compulsive traits found in childhood often clear up or respond promptly to treatment.
3. Some episodes are transitory and relatively circumscribed. Such patients frequently have a good prognosis if they undergo psychotherapy.

4. Unfortunately, many of these reactions have a tendency to become chronic and often follow a remitting course. As such, they are often resistant to treatment.
5. In general, the prognosis is more favorable when—
   a. The symptoms are of short duration.
   b. Environmental stressors are prominent.
   c. There is a good environment to return to following treatment.
   d. Interpersonal relationships are good.

F. Treatment
   1. Psychotherapy
      a. Intensive psychoanalytically oriented psychotherapy was at one time thought to be the treatment of choice. However, it would appear that only a small number of people with this disorder respond to such treatment.
      b. Supportive psychotherapy is often helpful. However, it should be kept in mind that responses to psychotherapy will often last only a matter of hours, and then the individual's doubts recur.
   2. Behavioral therapy
      a. Behavioral therapy has been tried recently. In this, the underlying complexities of the disorder are largely ignored, and attempts are made to focus on the person's behavior.
      b. The treatment is similar to behavioral treatment of phobias.
   3. Medications
      a. Anti-anxiety agents, neuroleptics, and antidepressant agents are sometimes useful in relieving some of the symptoms that accompany obsessive-compulsive disorders.
      b. However, none of the known psychotropic drugs relieves the underlying obsessive-compulsive disorder.
   4. Hospitalization
      Hospitalization may be indicated when ritualistic behavior becomes intense.
   5. Somatic therapy
      a. Electroshock therapy has been used, often with disappointing results.
      b. Prefrontal leukotomy has been performed on some patients who have chronic crippling disorders.

G. Case example

Mrs. B., a thirty-three-year-old housewife, consulted a psychiatrist, complaining of fear of germs and dirt, obsessions about religious ideas, and obsessions about the number 3. These symptoms had begun about three months earlier, following the birth of her second child. She had had a similar episode five years earlier, after her first child was born.

This had lasted about six months and finally cleared up during counselling with her pastor.

She was a bright person who was always orderly, methodical, conscientious, and dependable. As a child, she was overly concerned with the "normal" compulsions that children have, such as counting the pickets in fences and avoiding the cracks in sidewalk. At ten she became obsessed with the idea that she would die on a certain Tuesday in October.

In her present episode she had developed a number of compulsions in response to her fears and obsessions. For example, she washed her hands repeatedly and relaundered clothes because of her fear of germs and dirt, and she avoided reading automobile license plates and house numbers because she wished to avoid the number 3. After several weeks in the hospital, she improved enough so that she was able to carry on her housework, although she was still troubled somewhat by her symptoms.

In this case, note the previously compulsive personality and the typical obsessions and compulsions. In view of her compulsive personality and incomplete response to hospital treatment, one must be very cautious about prognosticating her future.

XI. Post-traumatic stress disorder [traumatic neurosis]
   A. Definition
   1. The essential feature is the development of characteristic symptoms after experiencing a psychologically traumatic event or events that is beyond the range of human experience usually considered normal (*DSM*-III).
   2. As defined here, the stressor producing this syndrome must be of sufficient magnitude to produce significant symptoms of distress in most individuals, and also outside the range of such common human experiences as simple bereavement, chronic illness, business losses, or marital conflict. Many different types of traumatic events have been noted to produce this syndrome. The trauma may be experienced alone (e.g., rape or assault) or in the company of groups of people (e.g., military combat). The traumatic events may be natural disasters (car accidents, airplane crashes, large fires) or man-made disasters (atomic bombing, torture, ambush, death camps) (*DSM*-III).
   B. Subtype
   Cases in which the symptoms last longer than six months after the onset or, in which the onset of symptoms occurs at least six months after the trauma (delayed) are listed as *post traumatic stress disorder, chronic, or delayed.*
   C. Characteristic symptoms
   Re-experiencing the traumatic event, numbing of responsiveness to, or involvement with, the external world, and a variety of other autonomic, dysphoric, or cognitive symptoms.
   D. Associated features
   Depression and anxiety are common.

E. Course
    1. May occur at any age.
    2. The symptoms may begin soon after the traumatic event or after a period of several days or even months.
    3. The more common course of this disorder is remission of the symptoms within six months after onset.

F. Predisposing factors
May include prior history of another mental disorder.

G. Prevalence
Unknown.

H. Treatment
    1. In general, treatment follows the principles set down for the other anxiety disorders.
    2. Early treatment seems to be essential to help resolve the condition.

References

American Psychiatric Association. *Diagnostic and Statistical Manual of Mental Disorders.* 3d ed. Washington, D. C., 1978–1979.

Bosselman, B. C. *Neurosis and Psychosis.* 3d ed. Springfield Ill.: Charles C Thomas, Publishers, 1964, chaps. 2, 3, 4, 5.

Eaton, M. T., Jr.; Peterson, M. H.; and David, J. M. *Psychiatry.* 3d ed. Flushing, N.Y.: Medical Examination Publishing Company, 1976, chap. 9.

Freedman, A. M.; Kaplan, H. I.; and Sadock, B. J. *Modern Synopsis of Comprehensive Textbook of Psychiatry.* Vol. 2. Baltimore: Williams & Wilkins Company, 1976, chap. 20.

Goodwin, D. W., and Guze, S. B. *Psychiatric Diagnosis.* 2d ed. New York: Oxford University Press, 1979, chaps. 3, 5, 6.

Kolb, L. C. *Modern Clinical Psychiatry.* 9th ed. Philadelphia: W. B. Saunders Company, 1977, chap. 22.

Nicholi, A. M., Jr., ed. *The Harvard Guide to Modern Psychiatry.* Cambridge: Belknap Press of Harvard University Press, 1978, chap. 10.

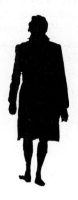

The mind has great influence over the body, and maladies often have their origin there.

Moliere, *Love's the Best Doctor* **(1665)**

Somatoform Disorders

I. Definition

The essential features of somatoform disorders are physical symptoms suggestive of physical disorder for which there is no demonstrable findings or known physiological mechanism but, instead, positive evidence or a strong presumption that the symptoms are linked to psychological factors or conflicts. The symptom production is not under voluntary control— *Diagnostic and Statistical Manual of Mental Disorders,* 3d edition (*DSM*-III).

II. Types

The categories of somatoform disorders are listed below. Each will be discussed in turn.

   A. Somatization disorder (Briquet's syndrome).

   B. Conversion disorder (or hysterical neurosis, conversion type)

   C. Psychogenic pain disorder

   D. Hypochondriasis (or hypochondriacal neurosis)

III. Somatization disorder

   A. Definition

      1. Somatization disorder is also known as Briquet's syndrome.

      2. The essential features are recurrent and multiple somatic complaints for which medical attention is sought but that are not apparently due to any physical disorder (*DSM*-III).

   B. Clinical symptoms

      1. Complaints are presented in a dramatic, vague, or exaggerated way, or as part of a complicated medical history. Some symptoms invariably refer to many organ systems; (e.g., gastrointestinal, female reproductive, cardiopulmonary, or psychosexual symptoms). Common physical complaints are headaches, fatigue, palpitations, fainting, nausea, vomiting, abdominal pains, bowel troubles, allergies, menstrual and sexual difficulties, and conversion symptoms. It is a chronic poly-symptomatic disorder.

      2. Often, it is difficult to determine when the illness started or why the patient sought medical examination.

      3. The conversion symptoms suggest neurological damage and are sometimes called *pseudoneurological* or *grand hysterical symptoms.*

      4. Virtually everyone experiences many somatic symptoms, but we do not complain of them and rarely report them to a physician when we are examined because we interpret the physician's questions as referring to "significant" symptoms.

   C. Associated features

   Anxiety and depression are extremely common. It may be the depression for which the individual seeks psychiatric treatment.

   D. Onset and courses

      1. Begins early in adult life (prior to age thirty).

      2. Rare in males.

3. Course is chronic but fluctuating.
4. Patients often have many medical examinations, are often admitted to hospitals for evaluation, and are frequently subjected to surgery.
5. The patients' lives are often dominated by their symptoms.
E. Case example

A forty-six-year-old married woman presented herself at a hospital with a twenty-year history of multiple physical complaints, especially abdominal pain, dating back fifteen years. Asked her reason for seeking hospitalization, she immediately recited a long list of physicians, hospitals, and clinics she had visited, underscoring her dissatisfaction with all of them. She was very dramatic in her presentation. Although sexual themes appeared to underlie her symptomotology and behavior, she focused entirely on her physical symptoms, especially those referrable to her abdomen. She reported that she had suffered for fifteen years and had continually sought medical care, and she stated, with a sort of glee, that all attempts had failed. Some of her physical symptoms were described in such a way that they seemed self-induced. For example, she said, "I was bleeding from the vagina, but I didn't pick at any *specific* place." In addition to seeing many internists, gastroenterologists, surgeons, gynecologists, and other specialists, she had seen several psychiatrists, who had attempted psychotherapy and psychotropic medication. A number of neurological examinations by excellent neurologists had been negative. A laproscopy had been essentially negative. All medication had been unsuccessful.

On psychiatric examination, she was overly dramatic and superficial. She rambled on about her symptoms and tried to control the interview. She focused entirely on her physical symptoms although there was a strong underlying sexual connotation.

After three or four weeks in the hospital, after attempts with various kinds of medication, psychotherapy, and joint therapy with her husband had failed, she left in an angry mood and proceeded to another hospital in a nearby city.

IV. Conversion disorder
A. Definition
1. Conversion disorder is also known as hysterical neurosis, conversion type.
2. The essential feature of conversion disorder is a clinical picture in which the predominant disturbance is a loss or alteration of physical functioning that suggests a physical disorder but that is actually a direct expression of psychological conflict or need. Psychological factors are judged causal because: (a) There is a temporal relationship between such factors and the development of the disorders; (b) The symptoms enable the individual to get support from the environment. The disturbance is not under voluntary control and not explained by any known physical disorder after appropriate examination.

3. Dynamically, it is a disorder in which unconscious conflict is manifested as disguised and symbolic somatic symptoms. That is, the anxiety arising out of some conflictual situation is converted into somatic symptoms in parts of the body innervated by the sensorimotor system (symbolic somatization). Thus, the conflict is reflected as physical symptoms instead of being expressed directly.

B. Differentiation from malingering

Conversion disorder must be distinguished from malingering.

    1. *Malingering* is conscious simulation of illness in order to avoid an unpleasant or intolerable alternative. Thus, there are two aspects:

        a. The voluntary production of symptoms suggesting physical disorder,

        b. An obvious recognizable environmental goal.

    2. The differentiation between conversion disorder and malingering is sometimes difficult because—

        a. Some behavior may be in part consciously determined and in part unconsciously determined.

        b. Many hysterical patients are so histrionic about their symptoms, and their secondary gain is so obvious, that one sees them as consciously feigning or simulating disease.

    3. Psychiatrists, however, should regard malingering as possibly indicative of some serious underlying psychopathology.

C. Prevalence

    1. Classical conversion disorder is less common than it was at the turn of the century.

    2. Conversion symptoms, however, are fairly common.

    3. Conversion elements are commonly seen in compensation cases.

    4. Conversion disorder is usually considered to be more common among women, although it is seen in men in the military setting.

    5. Classical conversion disorder is rarely seen in ordinary psychiatric practice, but is more commonly seen by neurologists, orthopedic surgeons, and by military physicians, especially in time of war.

D. Symptoms

    1. Somatic symptoms

        a. The somatic symptoms can vary widely. Frequently, they simulate organic disease and represent the patient's idea of the disease. The closeness with which the patient's symptoms approximate the symptoms of an organic disease depends in large measure on the patient's medical and psychological sophistication.

        b. The somatic symptoms chiefly involve organs that are in contact with the external world.

c. The distribution of the symptoms is unphysiological and non-anatomical.
d. Somatic symptoms can be considered under two headings:
   (1) Motor symptoms, such as convulsive states, paralysis, paresis (muscular weakness), or aphonia (inability to produce normal speech)
   (2) Sensory disturbances, such as analgesia (diminished sense of pain), anesthesia (absence of feeling), blindness, deafness, globus hystericus (sensation of lump in throat), or pain (most commonly abdominal).
2. Psychological symptoms
  a. The mental-status evaluation of the person with conversion disorder reveals no significant abnormalities.
  b. The classical psychological symptom in the conversion disorder is the patient's indifference to the illness (*la belle indifference*). Though the symptoms are obviously disabling, the patient seems unconcerned and shows no anxiety. However, it should be kept in mind that people with serious medical illnesses may also be indifferent.
  c. Some histories show a pre-existing histrionic personality disorder or dependent personality disorder (see the chapter, "Personality Disorders").
  d. This disorder is unique in the *DSM*-III classification because specific mechanisms are thought to account for it (see primary gain and secondary gain under Psychopathology, that follows).
  e. The onset or exacerbation of the symptoms almost always follows a psychologically meaningful environmental stimuli.
E. Historical conceptions of psychopathology
  1. Hippocrates believed that conversion disorder resulted from a wandering uterus.
  2. In the seventeenth century, hysteria was thought to be due to demoniacal possession.
  3. Charcot believed it was a genetic reaction that resulted in degeneration of the nervous system. He demonstrated that the hysterical symptoms could be produced and removed by hypnotic suggestion. (He also believed that normal people could not be hypnotized.)
  4. Janet introduced the concept of dissociated mental processes in the subconscious. He demonstrated that automatisms were of unconscious origin.
  5. Both Babinski and Bernheim believed that the symptoms resulted from suggestion. (Bernheim's extensive work with hypnosis led him to believe that normal people could be hypnotized.)

6. Breuer and Freud introduced the concept of repressed conflict as the source of conversion. Freud believed that the repressed conflict was the Oedipus complex.
7. Most authorities now feel that any highly charged instinct or impulse may be involved.

F. Psychopathology
1. Essentially, the psychopathology is repression of a conflict and conversion of the anxiety into a somatic symptom that is symbolic of the underlying conflict.
2. It was thought that only sexual conflict produced conversion symptoms. Theorists now believe that all types of instinctual impulses may find expression in this manner.
3. The premorbid personality is often histrionic. Such individuals are theatrical, shallow, superficial, or insincere. They are often narcissistic and manipulative. They go through the motions of feeling without really experiencing emotion and tend to overreact to minor stimuli.
4. The precipitating factor may seem trivial but have a special meaning to the person (thus, as in anxiety disorder, it is important to know the setting in which the first hysterical symptoms occurred).
5. The choice of symptom may be determined in several ways.
   a. Events may tend to focus the conflict in a specific area (e.g., a tonsillectomy or other type of operation on the throat or neck may be a precursor to aphonia that is an expression of some underlying conflict).
   b. The experience of the organ in relation to the conflict may be the determinant (e.g., paralysis of a hand with which the patient has struck someone in anger).
   c. The suitability of the organ to express the conflict symbolically may also dictate the choice (e.g., paralysis of the legs as a defense against meeting a threat by either attack or flight).
6. In conversion disorder, both primary gain and secondary gain are observed.
   a. The *primary gain* is the relief of anxiety.
   b. The *secondary gain* is the advantage that accrues to the patient by virtue of the illness. Secondary gain is often a factor in illness, both emotional and physical; however, it is most prominent in the conversion disorders.

G. Onset, course, and prognosis
1. A conversion disorder may prolong or exaggerate symptoms that originally resulted from physical illness.
2. Conversion symptoms may develop following an accident.

3. In acute cases—where the onset is abrupt and the duration of symptoms has been short—the prognosis is usually favorable when the patient is treated.
4. When the symptoms have been allowed to endure for a sustained period, the prognosis is less hopeful.
    a. In such cases, the *secondary gain* operates to decrease the individual's motivation to get well by giving up the symptoms.
    b. However, active treatment of someone who is well motivated is often successful.
5. *DSM*-III states that the course is unknown, but probably of short duration when the onset is abrupt.
6. Some studies have indicated that, in the long term, some individuals with "conversion symptoms" reveal an underlying neurologic disorder.
7. The relative maturity of the premorbid personality and the intensity of the underlying conflict are factors that must be evaluated in estimating the prognosis.
H. Treatment
    1. Psychotherapy
        a. Supportive psychotherapy, including emotional support, reassurance, and environmental modification, is the most common treatment.
        b. Long-term, intensive insight psychotherapy seems indicated in only a small number of the cases.
    2. Various forms of behaviorial therapy have been tried.
    3. Medicines
        Anti-anxiety agents or anti-depressant agents are sometimes used to relieve the anxiety and depression.
I. Case example

The twenty-six-year-old soldier previously mentioned in the chapter, "Adaptations to Anxiety," p. 49, developed paralysis of his right hand when firing for the first time on the rifle range. This was a defense against repressed hostility to his father, who had been physically abusive of his mother many times and who often abandoned the family for long periods. Upon the father's return home, shortly before the young man entered the service, he again threatened his wife. At that point, the young man stepped up to his father and said, "If you ever strike my mother again, I'll kill you." However, he had a very well-developed conscience and obviously would have trouble following through such a threat.

When he first reached the rifle range and saw the target over his gunsights, he recalled the incident and "saw" the face of his father. Because his conscience could not let him "kill" his father, his right hand became paralyzed, thus preventing him from expressing the strong hostile feelings he had for the father.

V. Psychogenic pain disorder
A. Definition
  1. The predominant disturbance is pain (usually severe and pro-
     longed) in the absence of adequate physical findings, not attrib-
     utable to any other mental or physical disorder or, out of
     proportion to the physical findings, and associated with evidence
     of psychological etiology (*DSM*-III). This disorder is also known
     as *psychalgia*.
  2. As in conversion disorder, psychological factors are involved:
     a. There is a temporal relationship between a psychologically
        meaningful environmental stimulus and the onset or exac-
        erbation of the pain.
     b. The pain enables the patient to avoid a noxious activity or
        gain support from the environment.
  3. Often, the pain enables the patient to effect some secondary gain.
B. Associated features
  1. The individual continues to seek out doctors to obtain relief of
     the pain despite repeated reassurance that he or she is physically
     and neurologically normal.
  2. The patient refuses to consider the role of the psychological fac-
     tors in the cause of the pain.
  3. There is sometimes a symbolic meaning to the pain, and a past
     history of conversion phenomena.
C. Treatment
  1. Any psychiatric treatment must necessarily be based on adequate
     physical, neurological, and laboratory examinations, to rule out
     the evidence of physical disease. These are also a prerequisite to
     establishing the patient's trust in the physician's assurances
     about the patient's physical state.
  2. Supportive psychotherapy is probably the most useful approach
     in the treatment of this condition.
  3. The judicious prescription of anti-anxiety agents and other psy-
     chotropic drugs, including tricyclics, for the appropriate symp-
     toms is also often necessary.
  4. The physician should be prepared to offer the patient an ongoing
     treatment plan.
D. Case example

Mrs. W was admitted to the hospital complaining of nervousness and
backache. Her difficulty had begun eight or nine years earlier, and her
nervousness and complaints of backache increased. She had seen many
doctors and taken many forms of medication. Her husband, who was
retired, did all the housework because she was in pain and lying down
most of the time. She progressively withdrew from society, did not want to
go anywhere, and seemed to cling to him continuously. Prior to the
disorder, she had been an outgoing, social, and competent person who

managed the home and its affairs in a good-spirited but moderately worrisome way.

The patient had always indulged her three children and, since they had attained maturity, had given and loaned them sizable amounts of money. The husband thought that the children had come to expect her financial assistance and to take it for granted. The patient's nervousness and backache began about the time the younger daughter married a man she did not approve of.

At the time of admission to the hospital, the patient seemed incapacitated. As it turned out, her backache had become aggravated because the son-in-law had embezzled money from the company he worked for. Mrs. W. repaid the debt by expending the inheritance she had received from a bachelor uncle.

Physical, orthopedic, and neurological examinations revealed nothing significant except an old compression fracture of the twelfth thoracic vertebra, which had healed. However, over the years, she had required medication for her nerves and various pain-relieving medications.

She has been followed for several years since the initial hospitalization, and she still recurrently complains of backache and continues to seek medical help from various doctors.

VI. Hypochondriasis
  A. Definition
      1. The predominant disturbance is an unrealistic interpretation of physical signs or sensations as abnormal, leading to a preoccupation with the fear of having a disease or a belief that one already has it (*DSM*-III).
      2. The term derives from the term for the subcostal abdominal region, the hypochondrium, which at one time was believed to be the seat or the origin of the disorder.
      3. It is now presumed to be of psychogenic origin.
      4. The hypochondriac is painfully aware of sensations that most people ignore. In general, he or she exaggerates their intensity and importance.
      5. The hypochondriac's somatic preoccupation precludes any concern with underlying feelings or conflicts.
  B. Symptoms
      1. Awareness and exaggeration of physical sensations that most others disregard.
      2. Sometimes the somatic preoccupation is really an obsessional symptom, representing displacement of anxiety onto the body itself.
      3. Sometimes the hypochondriacal symptoms are vague; at other times, they are organ-centered.
      4. Physical findings are absent.

C. Psychopathology

In general, hypochondriasis is considered a reaction to any kind of conflictual situation. Thus, it might be considered a reaction to sexual conflict, to repressed hostility, to disappointment, to failure, and so forth.

D. Course and prognosis

The course is usually a chronic one, although it may be intermittent.

E. Treatment

1. No specific treatment has been very effective.

2. Psychotherapy has had only limited value; the best results have been obtained when treatment has begun early.

3. When hypochondriasis is suspected, careful physical and laboratory examinations should be made to rule out any underlying physical disease. It is important to remember that a hypochondriacal person can develop a serious physical disease.

4. Medications of various kinds have been prescribed for symptomatic relief, including antianxiety agents for anxiety symptoms, antidepressants for any depressive features, and so forth. Drugs often have only temporary effects.

5. Environmental modification is occasionally helpful.

References

American Psychiatric Association. *Diagnostic and Statistical Manual of Mental Disorders.* 3d ed. Washington, D. C., 1978–1979.

Bosselman, B. C. *Neurosis and Psychosis.* 3d ed. Springfield, Ill.: Charles C Thomas, Publishers, 1964, chaps. 2, 3, 4, 5.

Eaton, M. T., Jr.; Peterson, M. H.; and David, J. A. *Psychiatry.* 3d ed. Flushing, N. Y.: Medical Examination, Publishing Company, 1976, chap. 9.

Freedman, A. M.; Kaplan, H. I.; and Sadock, B. J. *Modern Synopsis of Comprehensive Textbook of Psychiatry.* Vol. 2. Baltimore: Williams & Wilkins Company, 1976, chap. 20.

Goodwin, D. W., and Guze, S. B. *Psychiatric Diagnosis.* 2d ed. New York: Oxford University Press, 1979, chaps. 3, 4.

Kolb, L. C. *Modern Clinical Psychiatry.* 9th ed. Philadelphia: W. B. Saunders Company, 1977, chap. 20.

Nicholi, A. M., ed. *The Harvard Guide to Modern Psychiatry.* Cambridge: Belknap Press of Harvard University Press, 1978, chap. 10.

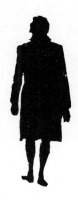

Not the power to remember,
But its very opposite,
The power to forget,
Is a necessary condition for our
    existence.

Shalom Asch, *The Nazarene*
(1939)

Dissociative Disorders (or Hysterical Neuroses, Dissociative Type)

I. Introduction

In previous classifications of mental illness, psychogenic amnesia and multiple personality were categorized as hysterical neurosis, dissociative type. They are now classified as dissociative disorders, which also include depersonalization disorder (formerly termed depersonalization neurosis), defined as a disorder in which the person has feelings of unreality, altered personality, or altered identity and might deny his or her own existence along with that of his environment.

Thus, the characteristic that is common to all the dissociative disorders is a constellation of recent mental events that is out of the patient's awareness but is capable, under certain conditions, of being brought into consciousness.

II. Definition

According to the *DSM*-III, the essential feature of these disorders is temporary alteration in the normally integrated functions of consciousness, identity, or motor behavior, so that some part of one or more of these functions is lost. Though the patients show gross personality disorganization, there are no indications of psychosis, although at times the disorder may be so diffuse as to appear psychotic. In these disorders there are alterations in the patient's state of consciousness or identity. The dissociation produces a demonstrable change in a person's behavior, feelings, or thoughts.

III. Psychopathology

A. Essentially, the disorder reflects the mechanism of dissociation—that is, the unconscious detachment of certain behavior or aspects of personality from the normal or usual patterns of an individual. The detached material then usually functions alone (compartmentalization).

B. It is a more massive type of forgetting than is seen in simple repression.

C. The ego is protecting itself against something that is critically dangerous and defending itself against overwhelming anxiety that develops because of an emotional bind.

D. Although the dissociation is handicapping, it relieves the individual's anxiety.

E. Dissociation is also symbolic and may have more than one meaning to the patient.

F. Primary gain (relief of anxiety) and secondary gain (advantage that accrues to the patient by virtue of the disorder) are evident in this condition (as they are in conversion disorders).

G. The premorbid person is said to be immature and egocentric and have experienced some type of episodic emotional disturbance early in life. Still others are said to be histrionic, schizoid, or passive.

IV. Types
A. Psychogenic amnesia
B. Psychogenic fugue
C. Multiple personality
D. Depersonalization disorder (or, Depersonalization neurosis)

V. Psychogenic amnesia
A. Definition

The essential feature is a sudden onset of a disturbance in the ability to recall important personal information registered and stored in memory, in the absence of an underlying organic mental disorder, or the traveling to another locale with the assumption of a new identity (*DSM*-III). See also the discussion of Dissociation in the chapter, "Adaptations to Anxiety."

B. There are four types of disturbance in recall.
1. Localized amnesia

Localized amnesia, failure to recall all events during a circumscribed period of time, is the most common type.
2. Selective amnesia

Selective amnesia is failure to recall some, but not all, the events that occurred during a circumscribed period of time.
3. Generalized amnesia

Generalized amnesia is failure to recall one's entire life.
4. Continuous amnesia

Continuous amnesia is failure to recall events subsequent to a specific time and up to, and including, the present.

C. Psychogenic amnesia is a pathological loss of memory.
1. This type of amnesia must be distinguished from the amnesias associated with organic brain damage and alcoholism.
2. It is more than a mere forgetting. Rather, it is an active "blotting out" of consciousness containing conflictual material.
3. It is most often a response to intense feelings such as terror, anger, or guilt.
4. Its onset is usually sudden, and it is of brief duration.
5. It is apparently rare and is usually seen in wartime or during natural disasters.
6. The individual is usually indifferent to the loss of memory (a similar indifference is found in conversion disorder).
7. Case example

Mrs. H., a forty-two-year-old housewife, entered the hospital complaining of several brief periods of memory loss. History revealed that the onset of the first episode coincided with her learning that her husband was going out with another woman. Subsequent episodes usually followed some incident in which she was reminded of the "other woman."

VI. Psychogenic fugue

A. The essential feature of the form of amnesia called *psychogenic fugue* is sudden and unexpected travel away from home or customary work locale and the assumption of a new identity and inability to recall one's prior identity, in the absence of an underlying organic mental disorder (*DSM*-III). Thus, it is dissociation characterized by loss of memory of life in the previous environment.

    1. During this changed state of consciousness, the individual operates on his or her unconscious strivings. In the fugue, these individuals often perform complicated activities and permit themselves to follow unconscious feelings, which their consciences ordinarily restrain them from doing. In a sense, the fugue state permits them to do a certain amount of "acting out."

    2. In addition, the individuals sometimes "lose" their identity by "forgetting" their names; at other times, they may "change" their identity by assuming a different name.

    3. They often appear quite normal to observers.

    4. Amnesia may follow the termination of the fugue.

    5. Prevalence

        a. It is apparently rare but more common in wartime or in times of natural disasters.

        b. The person who develops this disorder may use alcohol excessively.

    6. Case example

> J. R., a twenty-five-year-old soldier, was admitted to the prison ward of a military hospital, accused of desertion. His history revealed that he had served with distinction in combat and was twice wounded. Following his second wound, he was evacuated to the United States mainland for further treatment. After a brief period at one hospital, the medical staff decided he could be managed best at another hospital several hundred miles away and placed him on a train for that destination. The man never arrived at the second hospital. Six months later, he was discovered in another section of the country, living the life of a civilian under an assumed name. He was unable to identify himself correctly and could not account for his activities during the entire six-month period. His real identity was established only through his fingerprints.

VII. Multiple personality

A. Definition

The essential feature is the domination of the individual by one of two or more distinct personalities at any one time.

B. These two or more different personalities are separate and compartmentalized. In general, the primary character is proper and moral, and the secondary personality is hedonistic and impulse-ridden.

C. The transition from one personality to another is usually sudden.
D. Like the other dissociative states, it is rare. According to Nemiah, only a few more than a hundred cases have been described in the psychiatric literature in the last two hundred years, the great majority being reported between 1890 and 1920.
E. While dissociation is the major mechanism operating in this disorder, identification is also evident in the fashioning of the second personality.

VIII. Depersonalization disorder (or depersonalization neurosis)
A. Definition
  1. *Depersonalization disorder* involves an alteration in the perception or experience of the self so that the feeling of one's own reality is temporarily lost. This is manifested by a sense of self-estrangement or unreality, which may include the feeling that one's extremities have changed in size, or a sense of perceiving oneself from a distance (*DSM* -III).
  2. Or, it may be defined as a disorder of affect, in which the person has feelings of unreality, altered personality, or altered identity. Patients may deny their own existence or that of their environment.
  3. An essential feature is the frequent occurrence of prolonged episodes.
B. Depersonalization
  1. Depersonalization disorder is not to be confused with depersonalization, which occurs as a secondary finding in other disorders.
  2. Brief episodes of depersonalization are a common symptom, said to occur in 30 to 70 percent of young adults.
  3. Depersonalization is not considered an illness.
  4. Some common examples of depersonalization are hypnogogic hallucinations (the mental images that occur just before sleep) and hypnopompic hallucinations (images seen in dreams that persist on awakening). These are experienced by healthy people.
C. Types
  Related to depersonalization disorder, which is described in *DSM*-III as having a chronic, recurrent course with marked exacerbations and remissions, are the following:
  1. Trance states and trancelike states
    A *trance state* is a psychological stupor characterized by immobility and unresponsiveness to the environment. It usually has a sudden onset, and amnesia follows. A *trancelike state* is a similar experience, ordinarily induced in normal individuals by prolonged and unusual concentration on a task or object.

2. Feelings of unreality.
   a. *Feelings of unreality* are feelings that one is unreal.
   b. *Feelings of derealization* are feelings that the environment has changed.
   c. *Depersonalization* (see above) is a sense of estrangement from oneself.
3. *Déjà vu*
   Déjà vu is a subjective sensation that an experience that is really happening for the first time occurred on a previous occasion. Experienced by normal people, it also occurs in certain disorders, including psychotic disorders and in organic mental disorders.
4. Feelings of estrangement
   Feelings of estrangement are a sense of detachment from people, the environment, or concepts. The term embraces *paramnesia*, distortion or falsification of memory in which the individual confuses reality and fantasy.
5. Fascination, or fixation
   Fascination, or *fixation,* is a trancelike state induced in individuals (e.g., pilots) who are compelled to focus on a given object for long periods of time.
6. Cosmic consciousness, or illumination
   Cosmic consciousness, or *illumination,* is a fabulous sense of joy or well-being, sometimes produced by hallucinogenic drugs.
D. Course and prognosis
   1. The course and prognosis depend upon the patient's motivation to get well, his or her ego-strength, the duration of the reaction, and the strength of the secondary gain.
   2. According to *DSM*-III, depersonalization disorder is considered to have a chronic course.
   3. The symptoms of all the dissociative disorders usually increase when the patient is confronted with mounting anxiety.
   4. In general, the immediate prognosis is good when the dissociative episode has an acute onset.
   5. When there is a close relationship between some environmental factor and the onset, the prognosis is good if the person is removed from the threatening environment.
   6. In some cases, the long-term prognosis is only fair.
E. Treatment
   1. The treatment should be dynamic or psychoanalytically oriented psychotherapy.
   2. See the treatments listed under Conversion disorders in the chapter "Somatoform Disorders."

References

American Psychiatric Association. *Diagnostic and Statistical Manual of Mental Disorders*. 3d ed. Washington, D.C., 1978–1979.

Eaton, M. T., Jr.; Peterson, M H.; and Davis, J. A. *Psychiatry*. 3d ed. Flushing, N. Y.: Medical Examination Publishing Company, 1976, chap. 9.

Freedman, A. M.; Kaplan, H. I.; and Sadock, B. J. *Modern Synopsis of Comprehensive Textbook of Psychiatry*. Baltimore: Williams & Wilkins Company, 1976, chap. 20.

Kolb, L. C. *Modern Clinical Psychiatry*. 9th ed. Philadelphia: W. B. Saunders Company, 1977, chap. 20.

Nemiah, John. In A. M. Nicholi (Ed.), *The Harvard Guide to Modern Psychiatry*, chapter 10. Cambridge: Belknap Press of Harvard University Press, 1978.

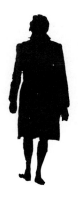

We are never so easily deceived as when we imagine we are deceiving others.

La Rochefoucauld: *Maxims* **(1665)**

Factitious Disorders

I. Introduction

A. Factitious disorders are a new classification in the *Diagnostic and Statistical Manual of Mental Disorders,* 3d edition (*DSM*-III). It encompasses those factitious (or pseudo; unnatural) conditions that are produced by individuals, are under voluntary control, and do not appear goal-directed.

B. Thus, factitious disorders are distinguished from conversion disorders, on the one hand, and malingering, on the other.

C. In previous classifications, some of these disorders were considered forms of hysteria.

II. Types

Factitious disorders may be characterized by (1) psychological symptoms; or (2) by physical symptoms.

III. Factitious disorder with psychological symptoms

A. Definition

1. The essential feature is a voluntary production of symptoms suggestive of mental disorder, in the absence of malingering.

2. This disorder was formerly diagnosed as *Ganser syndrome,* and is sometimes called the *nonsense syndrome* or *prison psychosis.*

B. It is commonly employed by those who seek to mislead others about their true emotional state. It is characterized by childish, ludicrous behavior.

C. The individual's replies or responses are approximate, *"vorbeireden."* Hence, it is sometimes called the *syndrome of approximate answers.*

D. It may be superimposed on another mental disorder. For example, an individual who has been hospitalized for a schizophrenic disorder may, upon learning that he or she is about to be discharged, simulate a new bizarre symptom or a past one.

IV. Factitious disorder with physical symptoms (Münchausen syndrome)

A. Definition

The essential feature of this disorder is the individual's plausible presentation of factitious physical symptoms of such severity that he or she is able to obtain and sustain many hospitalizations (*DSM*-III).

B. Character of the disorder

1. Persons with this disorder can present and simulate illness of virtually any type. Originally it was thought that such patients fell into one of four categories:

   a. The acute abdominal type
   b. The neurological type
   c. The hemorrhagic type
   d. The cutaneous type.

2. It is now thought that the clinical picture is limited only by the individual's medical sophistication and imagination.

C. From a psychodynamic point of view, the patient seems to be seeking a repetitive relationship with a physician to reenact a maternal type of relationship.

D. This is a rare disorder and difficult to treat.

References

American Psychiatric Association. *Diagnostic and Statistical Manual of Mental Disorders.* 3d ed. Washington, D. C., 1978–1979.

Kolb, L. C. *Modern Clinical Psychiatry.* 9th ed. Philadelphia: W. B. Saunders Company, 1977, chap. 22.

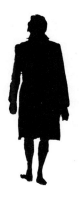

I find, by experience, that the mind
and the body are more than married,
For they are most intimately united;
And when the one suffers, the other
sympathizes.

**Philip T. Stanhope, 4th Earl of
Chesterfield (1694-1773)**

Psychological Factors Affecting Physical Condition (Psychophysiologic Disorders)

I. Introduction

A. In the Third Edition of the *Diagnostic and Statistical Manual,* there is no category labelled Psychophysiologic or Psychosomatic Disorders. Instead, there is a classification of Psychological Factors Affecting Physical Condition. This provides for classifying those physical conditions either with demonstrable organic pathology (such as rheumatoid arthritis), or a known pathophysiological process (such as migraine headache) which show evidence of a temporal relationship to psychologically meaningful environmental stimuli in the initiation, exacerbation, or maintenance of the physical symptoms.

B. In this chapter, I shall describe those disorders which in the past have, and continue to be, regarded as psychosomatic and about which much has been written in the psychiatric literature.

C. Thus, the topics in this chapter now include: (1) the traditional psychosomatic disorders; (2) any disorder that would have been diagnosed as psychophysiologic disorder by the criteria of *DSM*-II; and (3) any physical condition in which psychological factors are significant in the onset, exacerbation, or perpetuation of the disorder.

II. Definition

According to *A Psychiatric Glossary,* 1980, psychophysiologic disorders are "a group of disorders characterized by physical symptoms that are caused by emotional factors and that involve a single organ system, usually under *autonomic nervous system* control. Symptoms are caused by physiological changes that normally accompany certain emotional states, but in these disorders the changes are more intense and sustained. Frequently called *psychosomatic* disorders. These disorders are usually named and classified according to the organ system involved (e.g., gastrointestinal, respiratory)."[1]

III. The role of conflict

A. There are four schools of thought regarding the specificity of conflict in the psychosomatic disorders. All address the relationship between stress and the onset or course of the disorder and the question of whether or not specific types of stress produce specific psychosomatic states.

B. Hypotheses
   1. The specificity model
      Adherents of *specificity* believe that the psychological factors that produce a particular type of disorder are specific and symbolic. So far, no studies have offered conclusive proof of this

---

1. Definition from *A Psychiatric Glossary,* 5th ed., American Psychiatric Association, Washington, D.C., 1980.

model; the only current evidence is the relationship between the behavior of individuals with Type A personality and the development of coronary heart disease.

   2. The nonspecific model
      Adherents of *nonspecifity* believe that many different psychological factors may produce a given disorder, the nature of the response being dependent upon constitutional factors and the acquired vulnerability of the organ. This model is consistent with some of the current research findings.
   3. The individual-response specificity model
      Proponents of *individual-response specificity* hold that a specific constellation of psychological factors, plus a local somatic vulnerability, produce a particular psychosomatic disorder. This theory takes into account both local vulnerability and psychogenic specificity.
   4. The body-image perception model
      Proponents of the theory of *body-image perception* believe that one's body image determines the illness or symptom that one develops in response to stress. Body image does seem to be a factor in obesity and anorexia nervosa (see the following).

IV. Psychosomatic gastrointestinal reactions

   A. Most everyone is aware of the relationship between emotions and the gastrointestinal tract. It is thought by many that food is, very early on, associated with feelings of security, attention, and love. Various types of psychosomatic disturbances are associated with eating, digesting, and eliminating food.
   B. Anorexia nervosa
      1. Definition
         A disorder marked by servere and prolonged refusal to eat with severe weight loss, amenorrhea or impotence, disturbance of body image and an intense fear of becoming obese. Most frequently encountered in girls and young women. May be associated with bulimia. Classified as an Eating disorder in *DSM-III*.[2]
      2. Description
         a. At one time, it was assumed that only females suffered from this disturbance, but about 10 percent of the patients are males.
         b. The cause of the illness is unknown.
         c. It is characterized by Goodwin et al. as "the relentless pursuit of thinness."

2. Definition from *A Psychiatric Glossary,* 5th ed., American Psychiatric Association, Washington, D.C., 1980.

d. It must be distinguished from other illnesses that are accompanied by weight loss, such as endocrine and other organic illnesses that produce malnutrition, loss of appetite, and loss of weight.

e. Clinical picture[3]
   (1) Refusal to maintain body weight over the normal minimum for one's age and height.
   (2) Loss in weight of 25 percent; or, if under eighteen years of age, a 25 percent loss in weight when the gain in weight projected from pediatric growth charts is added.
   (3) Disturbance of body image and inability to perceive body size accurately.
   (4) Intense fear of becoming obese that does not diminish as weight is lost.
   (5) There is no known medical illness to account for the loss of weight.
   (6) Amenorrhea.

f. Not all patients suffer a loss of appetite; some resist eating food despite being hungry.

g. Essentially, the behavior of the person with this illness is governed by the desire to lose weight and the intense fear of gaining it. The behavior includes marked dietary limitation; abuse of laxatives or diuretics or both; and, sometimes, self-induced vomiting.

h. The individual often seems unusually active for one who has lost so much appetite and weight.

3. Treatment
Treatment is far from satisfactory and there is no agreement about the best form.

a. Hospitalization
Some patients require constant observation in a locked psychiatric ward and tube feeding.

b. Medicine
Others have been successfully treated with phenothiazines.

c. Behavioral therapy
Techniques of behavioral modification have been used, and some success has been reported.

C. Obesity
1. Description
a. With rare exceptions, obesity results from overeating.
b. Many obese individuals overeat when they are emotionally upset.

---

3. Adapted from K. A. Halmi, "Anorexia Nervosa: Recent Investigation," *Annual Review of Medicine.* 29:137–148.

c. No studies find a specific personality type or psychodynamic conflict, although many clinicians consider the overeater to be orally fixated and dependent.
d. Patterns of overeating vary
   (1) The "binge" type engages in sudden compulsive ingestion of large amounts of food in a short period of time.
   (2) The "night-eating" type has anorexia in the morning and hyperphagia and insomnia in the evening.
   (3) Both types are said to be anxious and self-condemnatory after overeating.
e. Some obese people have a disturbed body image and view their body with loathing or contempt.

2. Course and prognosis
   a. The likelihood of sustained weight loss is poor.
   b. Many patients are able to manage weight reduction for brief periods but, in general, their course is toward a progressive gain in weight.

3. Treatment
   a. Reduction of weight
      Weight reduction, in itself, does not usually produce lasting results.
   b. Medicines
      Anorexiants, mostly amphetamines or amphetamine-like substances, are prescribed. When used in conjunction with a supervised treatment program, including a diet, they have some limited value.
   c. Exercise
      Physical exercise is often recommended.
   d. Psychoanalytically oriented psychotherapy
      The results have been disappointing. However, patients with disturbed body images and the binge eating type seem to have responded to dynamically oriented psychotherapy.
   e. Group therapy
      Group therapy has had good results. Among the self-help groups are TOPS (Take off Pounds Sensibly) and Weight Watchers.
   f. Surgery
      The gastric by-pass procedure has become a treatment of choice among people whose obesity is severe and who have not responded to other treatment. There are hazards in a surgical approach, however, that should be considered before resorting to it.

g. Behavioral modification

This technique has been helpful but does not seem to solve the problem.

D. Peptic ulcer disease

1. Introduction

a. Peptic ulcer is regarded as a disease of civilization. It is more prevalent in urban areas and much more common among men than women. It was, however, more common in women before the 20th century.

b. It is usually considered a stress-related disorder.

2. Theories

a. In 1938, Alexander et al. described what they regarded as the conflict between oral-receptive tendencies (the wish to be taken care of) and a striving for independence. They believed that the oral tendencies and fantasies produced continuous gastric secretion that led to ulcer formation.

b. In 1953, Mahl and Karpe found that all the "high acid hours" were related to periods of high anxiety and that "the low acid hours" were related to low anxiety periods. The finding did not support the specificity theory but rather indicated that the anxiety, whatever its origin, increased the secretion of hydrochloric acid and susceptibility to peptic ulcer disease.

c. Many investigators believe in the importance of dependent-independent conflict, which is sometimes related in part to difficulties occurring during the early oral period. In addition, the tendency to be a "hypersecretor" of hydrochloric acid may be biologically or genetically common. Thus, according to Mirsky, a peptic ulcer forms "in response to meaningful life situations which mobilizes or intensifies this psychic conflict." (Mirsky, 1958)

3. Treatment

a. Psychotherapy does not eliminate the underlying predisposing factors (genetic factors and vulnerability).

b. Supportive psychotherapy might be helpful in assisting the ulcer bearer to cope better with the stresses of life that can aggravate the disease.

c. Perhaps the supportive relationship of the primary physician is as good as any.

E. Irritable bowel

1. Definition

This is a functional bowel disorder characterized by periods of diarrhea alternating with periods of constipation, abdominal cramps, and flatulence, and sometimes by increased mucus in the stool.

2. Theories
   a. Stress is an important aggravating factor in this illness.
   b. Some authorities feel such patients are typically obsessive-compulsive in their personality makeup.
   c. Others point out that good empirical data to support this contention are not available.

F. Ulcerative colitis
  1. Definition
   Ulcerative colitis is an acute and chronic disease of the mucosa and submucosa of the colon. Bleeding, diarrhea, and abdominal cramps are typical symptoms.
  2. Etiology
   a. Despite much study, the etiology and pathogenesis remain obscure.
   b. There is some evidence for genetic factors, since it tends to occur in families.
   c. Emotional disturbances seem to be of some importance, at least as contributory.
   d. The ulcerative colitis patient has been described as dependent, indecisive, overly conscientious, aggressive, and hostile, although outwardly he or she may seem self-deprecating.
  3. Treatment
   a. At this time, there is no evidence that intensive psychotherapy is helpful in decreasing the symptoms of this disorder.
   b. Again, as with the ulcer patient, the supportive approach in helping the patient cope with the illness and stresses of life seems the most appropriate treatment.

G. Crohn's disease
  1. Crohn's disease is also known as *granulomatous enteritis and colitis.*
  2. There are many similiarities between these patients and those with ulcerative colitis.
  3. The patients are also said to have obsessive-compulsive traits.

V. Psychosomatic cardiovascular reactions
A. Introduction
  1. Most emotional reactions, including fear, anxiety, anger, elation, and excitement, are accompanied by cardiovascular changes.
  2. In addition, such feelings can aggravate existing cardiovascular disease and may lead to disturbances in rate and rhythm in patients with a constitutional predisposition to cardiac disease.

3. The presence of cardiovascular diseases (such as myocardial infarction, hypertension, or angina) may themselves produce various emotional states.

B. Coronary artery disease

1. Early studies that described coronary-disease-prone personalities as compulsive, competitive, and hard driving have not been supported by subsequent reviews and research.

2. Although the issue of personality type in this disease is controversial, Rosenman and Freedman described a behavioral group (Type A) that they believe is prone to the development of coronary artery disease. Such a group is characterized by—

   a. Excessive competitive drive.
   b. Ambitiousness and achievement orientation.
   c. A chronic sense of urgency.
   d. An inclination to make multiple commitments.
   e. An immersion in deadlines.

C. Essential hypertension

1. Definition

   This is a systemic reaction in which there is a sustained elevation of blood pressure above 140/90 in the absence of any demonstrable pathology.

2. Etiology

   a. The etiology is incompletely understood.
   b. It is probably caused by an interplay of multiple factors.
   c. Previous studies that indicated that the hypertensive person was one who struggled continuously against hostile and aggressive impulses, but who was outwardly affable and easygoing, have not been substantiated.
   d. However, most clinicians believe that stress does have an important influence on the clinical course and on the possibility that complications will develop.

3. Treatment

   a. There is no good evidence that psychotherapy, biofeedback, or conditioning will permanently lower elevated blood pressure.
   b. So far, the anti-hypertensive medications are the important aspect of treatment.

D. Vasodepressor syncope

1. Definition

   This is a fainting due to acute peripheral circulatory inadequacy (with a sudden drop in blood pressure) that is quickly reversible.

2. It may occur in response to anxiety, pain, or shock.

3. The onset usually occurs while the individual is standing in the erect position and is commonly preceded by anxiety, including sweating, nausea, restlessness, muscle weakness, pallor, and sighing.
4. Psychophysiologically, it appears that the individual is preparing for action (fight or flight), but neither action occurs. Attacks are more apt to occur if fear is being denied.
E. Congestive heart failure
1. Anxiety imposes a burden, comparable to that of exertion, on the heart.
2. Stress often precipitates episodes of congestive heart failure.
F. Migraine headaches
1. This is a syndrome characterized by recurrent, severe unilateral headache (cephalgia), nausea, vomiting, and certain prodromal disturbances (scotoma, paresthesia, or speech difficulty).
2. The physiological mechanism has been described by H. G. Wolff. In brief, it is a vasoconstriction followed by a compensatory vasodilatation in the meningeal arteries, usually of one side only. It is this compensatory vasodilatation which is followed by pain.
3. Many different personality types have been described as specific to migraine patients.
4. As with other descriptions of this type, controls have been inadequate.
5. Most clinicians agree, however, that emotional stress may precipitate an attack in an individual vulnerable to migraine.
6. Treatment
a. Medications are of chief value in this disorder.
b. If stress is an aggravating factor, psychotherapy may be helpful.
c. Biofeedback has been used.

VI. Psychosomatic respiratory disorders
A. Various emotions such as hostility, anxiety, fear, or excitement may lead to disturbances in respiration.
B. The respiratory system is involved in one's earliest significant interpersonal relationships and is one of the earliest ways of expressing emotional reactions and needs.
C. Hyperventilation syndrome
1. Definition
a. This is a condition in which the individual is subject to repeated forced respirations, yawning, sensations of hunger for air, occasional tetany, chest pain, lightheadedness, paresthesias of the hand, feet, and face, and an intense conviction of impending death.

b. It is also known as the *effort syndrome,* or *neurocirculatory asthenia* (NCA).
c. Some authorities feel that the hyperventilation syndrome is probably the least recognized anxiety disorder.
2. The individual often does not realize that he or she is over-breathing.
3. Oftentimes the individual is able to describe the conditions in which the attacks occur. Sometimes they are associated with disturbing dreams.
4. The hyperventilation syndrome may develop in situations other than emotional stress (e.g., in certain febrile illnesses; at high altitudes).
5. Widely divergent emotional states (e.g., fear, anxiety, grief, joy) may lead to hyperventilation. In most instances the reaction is out of proportion to the actual stress.
6. The person who hyperventilates is usually preoccupied with physical health.
7. There is no highly specific dynamic conflict which leads to this condition; rather, conflicts may be in many different areas.
8. The physiological changes accompanying hyperventilation explain most of its symptoms. (Alkalosis, which produces cerebral vasal constriction and a decreased cerebral blood flow.)
9. Treatment
   a. Psychotherapy has been helpful.
   b. Anti-anxiety agents and antidepressants have also been helpful.
   c. Another method is to have the patient hyperventilate and produce the physiological effects, then assist the patient to see the relationship between the disorder and the symptoms.

D. Asthma
   1. Definition
   This is an allergic disorder with dyspnea and wheezing due to bronchial obstruction resulting from bronchial spasm, bronchial edema, and mucus plugs.
   2. A specific etiology has not been isolated. The cause most thoroughly investigated has been hypersensitivity to allergens.
   3. Personality studies have indicated a wide range of personality types and have not identified a particular conflict constellation.
   4. Emotional upsets can aggravate the condition.
   5. Tricyclic antidepressants have a bronchodilatory effect.

VII. Psychosomatic musculoskeletal disorders
A. There are various types of psychosomatic musculoskeletal disorders.
   1. Functional backache is often concerned in industrial accidents and compensation cases.

2. Tension headache
   a. Tension headache is most commonly related to chronic anxiety.
   b. There is no specific personality type associated with tension headaches.
   c. Headaches are common symptoms after a head injury and may persist for many months.
3. Rheumatoid arthritis
   a. Some observers have reported that the onset or aggravation of rheumatoid arthritis is related to a period of stress.
   b. Chronic tension and muscular contraction may cause impaired circulatory and articular changes.
   c. Although stress may initiate or aggravate the disease, no definite relationship between psychosomatic factors and the disease has been established.

VIII. Psychosomatic skin disorders
A. Blushing from embarassment and blanching with fear are commonly observed skin responses.
B. Many types of feelings—such as anger, guilt, tension, or erotic arousal—may lead to itching and subsequent scratching.
C. A wide variety of stresses may cause various dermatological disorders to flare up.
D. Hyperhidrosis can be produced by an increase in sweat secretion, which can be produced by fear or anxiety. Such sweating appears primarily in the axillae, the soles of the feet and the palms.

IX. Emotional reaction to physical illness
A. Apart from the disorders already mentioned, there are many illnesses in which the patient's psychological reaction may be important.
B. The patient's personality makeup and emotional needs should be taken into account in the treatment of any illness.
C. Examples of the psychological import of physical illness
   1. A fourteen-year-old boy became depressed when he learned that he had diabetes. Underlying the depression was the feeling that the diabetes was a punishment for masturbation.
   2. A twenty-eight-year-old woman had been an invalid since sixteen, when she first developed rheumatic heart disease. Although her heart disease was sufficient to restrict her activity somewhat, her invalidism (regression) was out of proportion to the damage to her heart valve. Rehabilitation, in this instance, was focused mainly on her emotional reaction to the physical illness.
D. It should be kept in mind that whatever a person's particular illness may be, there is usually accompanying anxiety; this anxiety must be recognized and treated.

References

Alexander, F.; French, T. M.; and Pollack, G. A. *Psychosomatic Specifity: Experimental Study and Results.* Chicago: University of Chicago Press, 1968.

American Psychiatric Association. *A Psychiatric Glossary.* Washington, D. C., 1980.

————. *Diagnostic and Statistical Manual of Mental Disorders.* 3d ed. Washington, D. C., 1978–1979.

Eaton, M. T., Jr.; Peterson, M. H.; and Davis, J. A. *Psychiatry.* 3d ed. Flushing, N. Y.: Medical Examination Publishing Company, 1976, chap. 8.

Freedman, A. M.; Kaplan, H. I.; and Sadock, B. J. *Modern Synopsis of Comprehensive Textbook of Psychiatry.* Vol. 2. 2d ed. Baltimore: Williams & Wilkins Company, 1976.

Goodwin, Donald W., and Guze, Samuel B. *Psychiatric Diagnosis.* 2d ed. New York: Oxford University Press, 1979. chap. 11.

Kirsner, J. B., and Palmer, W. L. "Ulcerative Colitis." *Journal of the American Medical Association* 155 (1954): 341.

Kolb, L. C. *Modern Clinical Psychiatry.* 9th ed. Philadelphia: W. B. Saunders Company, 1977, chap. 23.

Mahl, G. S., and Karpe, R. "Emotions and Hydrochloric Acid Secretion During Psychoanalytic Hours." *Psychomatic Medicine* 15 (1953): 312–327.

Mirsky, I. A. "Physiologic, Psychologic and Social Determinants in the Etiology of Duodenal Ulcer." *American Journal of Digestive Diseases* 285 (1958).

Nicholi, A. M., ed. *Harvard Guide to Modern Psychiatry.* Cambridge: Belknap Press of Harvard University Press, 1978, chap. 16.

Rosenman, R. H., and Friedman, M. "Behavior Patterns, Blood Lipids and Coronary Heart Disease." *Journal of the American Medical Association* 184:934–938.

————. "Coronary Heart Disease in the Western Collaborative Group Study." *Journal of the American Medical Association* 223, no. 8: 872–877.

Wolff, H. G. *Headache and Other Head Pain.* New York: Oxford University Press, 1963.

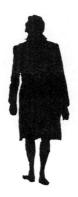

There is something in the character of every man which cannot be altered: It is the skeleton of his character. Trying to change it is like trying to train sheep to pull a car.

G. C. Lichtenberg: *Reflections* **(1799)**

Personality Disorders

I. Definition

These disorders are characterized by deeply ingrained, inflexible, maladaptive patterns of relating to, perceiving, and thinking about the environment and oneself that are of sufficient severity to cause either significant impairment in adaptive functioning or subjective distress. Thus, they are pervasive personality traits and are exhibited in a wide range of important social and personal contexts. The manifestations of personality disorders are generally recognizable by the time of adolescence or earlier and continue throughout most of adult life, although they often become less obvious in middle or old age (*DSM*-III).

   A. Synonyms are character disorders; social deviants.

II. Personality development

   A. Personality is the sum total of a person's internal and external patterns of adjustment to life.

   B. Although there may be some variation in a person's behavior, the individual's adjustment is generally in a state of equilibrium because he or she has accumulated a repertoire of problem-solving techniques during growth and development.

   C. Personality reflects those coping mechanisms and ego defenses that one uses to maintain emotional equilibrium.

   D. It also reflects the compromise that one has made among the pressures from:
      1. Instinctual drives
      2. The environment
      3. The superego.

   E. Thus, personality usually reflects the individual's techniques of getting along with other people and results from early developmental factors, including the influences of society, culture, and childrearing patterns.

   F. Certain well-developed personality traits such as compulsiveness, narcissism, or dependency may be so minimal that they do not interfere with the individual's functioning.

III. Characteristics of personality disorder

   A. Individuals with personality disorders do not develop symptoms that bother them. In psychoanalytic terminology, they have a *character neurosis* rather than a *symptom neurosis.*

   B. The personality disorder is characterized by its lifelong nature and the person's repetitive, maladaptive, and often self-defeating behavior (rather than discomfort or physical and psychological symptoms).

   C. The disorders usually begin in childhood or adolescence and persist throughout most of adult life.

   D. People with personality disorders are usually anxiety-free except when they are confronted with environmental stress.

E. Because problems are expressed in a maladaptive form of living rather than in symptoms, it is rare for character-disordered individuals to seek help at their own initiative. In general, such people tolerate stress poorly. If they are confronted by minor stresses, they are apt to become anxious; if confronted by moderate stresses, they may develop transient psychotic reactions.

F. It should be remembered that many of the difficulties people have adjusting to the world may be due to social stress or disarrangement rather than to disordered character.

G. When the occupation or environment accepts or rewards the individual's behavior, such personality patterns may be compatible with success and satisfaction. For example, a narcissistic person might be very successful in the entertainment world.

IV. **Etiological factors**

Among the possible causal factors are:

A. Constitutional predisposition

B. Childhood experiences that have fostered deviant behavior—
  1. Being rewarded for "acting-out" behavior (such as temper tantrums or hostile-aggressive behavior).
  2. Being encouraged when overly conforming and being discouraged when creative.
  3. Circumstances in which normal behavior is not allowed to develop, e.g., having a rigid, unreasonable parent who adamantly refuses to accept any reason for nonconformity.

C. Identification with parents or other authority figures who have similar deviancies.

V. **Types of personality disorders**

A. Included under this classification are
  1. Paranoid personality disorder
  2. Schizoid (introverted) personality disorder
  3. Schizotypal personality disorder
  4. Histrionic personality disorder
  5. Narcissistic personality disorder
  6. Antisocial personality disorder
  7. Borderline personality disorder
  8. Avoidant personality disorder
  9. Dependent personality disorder
  10. Compulsive personality disorder
  11. Passive-aggressive personality disorder

B. In the new multiaxial classification of *DSM*-III, these disorders are listed under Axis II.

C. The definitions of the personality disorders discussed in the rest of this chapter are based on the descriptions in *DSM*-III.

VI. Paranoid personality

A. Definition

People with this personality disorder exhibit a pervasive and long-standing suspiciousness and mistrust of people, hypersensitivity, hypervigilance, unwarranted suspicions, jealousy, envy, an excessive feeling of self-importance, and a tendency to blame others and ascribe evil motives to them. They are regarded by others as hostile, stubborn, and defensive. They may be litigious.

B. Features

1. Persons with paranoid personalities rarely seek psychiatric treatment on their own.
2. The disorder is more common in men.
3. Most paranoid people avoid intimacy.

C. Etiology

1. See Etiological factors.
2. Some think that paranoid personalities often have parents of the opposite sex who are domineering, overprotective, and ambivalent, and parents of the same sex who are submissive, passive and, as Freedman et al. wrote, relatively unavailable to the child "as an object for identification."

D. Case example

J. H., a thirty-eight-year-old married man, was referred to the court's psychiatric consultant for evaluation after he had pleaded guilty to a charge of assault growing out of a complaint filed by his wife, whom he had beaten up one evening in a bar.

He admitted to one previous court appearance for leaving the scene of an accident and also admitted to being jailed overnight once for drunkenness. In an interview, he admitted to having beaten his wife once previously, but said that he only slapped her with his open hand. He admitted to arguing with his wife but claimed the arguments were not too different from those most married couples have.

His wife reported that he carried a chip on his shoulder most of the time and felt that people owed him something. She indicated that he was "very suspicious" of her friends and that he would not talk to them. He constantly suspected that his wife was unfaithful and was unable to place any trust and confidence in physicians even though, by neglecting to do so, he had impaired his health. His Minnesota Multiphasic Personality Inventory profile was consistent with a diagnosis of paranoid personality. He seemed to be the sort of person who could keep his paranoid feelings under control as long as he did not drink. When he drank, his suspicions and projected feelings were enhanced, and he acted on them.

VII. Schizoid personality
A. Definition
  1. Also known as *introverted personality*.
  2. The essential features of the *schizoid personality* are a defect in the capacity to form social relationships, introversion, and bland or constricted affect. People with this disorder often show little desire for social involvement, are reserved, withdrawn, seclusive, and pursue solitary interests or hobbies. They seem unable to express aggressiveness or hostility and often appear cold, aloof, and distant. Autistic thinking and day dreaming are common. They appear self-absorbed.
B. Predisposing factor
  Introverted personality disorder of childhood.
C. Case example

C. N., a twenty-five-year-old single woman, was referred to the court's psychiatric consultant for evaluation after she had been arrested in the lobby of a downtown hotel for drunkenness. Aside from her drunken state, no behavioral disturbance had brought her to the attention of the authorities. She had never been arrested previously.

During the interview, she was very quiet. Most of the information obtained from her was through a question-and-answer approach. She responded to direct questions, but volunteered very little about herself. She had a somewhat disheveled appearance and wore an unusual amount of cheap jewelry. Although she was a college graduate, she was working as a cocktail waitress in one of the local country clubs. She readily admitted to having a drinking problem and estimated that about twice a month she drank to the point of blacking out. Most of her drinking was done alone, although some of it was in the company of other waitresses. She did not seem to be very introspective or reflective. When asked to give her opinion of herself, she said that she never thought much about herself. She admitted to being very passive and said that she felt easily led. She admitted to feelings of inferiority and did not plan for the future. The probation officer who had investigated her reported that she was a very shy, withdrawn person, sadly lacking in self-confidence.

VIII. Schizotypal personality
A. This is a new classification in *DSM*-III.
B. This group includes some persons who, in the past, may have been diagnosed as schizoid personalities, simple schizophrenics, or borderline schizophrenics.
C. Definition
  The essential features are various oddities of thinking, perception, communication, and behavior, never severe enough to meet the criteria for schizophrenia. The disturbance in thinking may be expressed as magical thinking, ideas of reference, or paranoid idea-

tion. The perceptual disturbances may include recurrent illusions, depersonalization, or derealization. Communication disturbances may be manifested as odd or unclear expression of concepts, but not to the point of derailment (loosening of association) or incoherence. Speech may be tangential, overelaborate, or circumstantial. Frequently, the behavioral manifestations include social isolation and constricted or inappropriate affect (*DSM*-III).

D. Associated features
   1. Frequently, there are varying mixtures of anxiety, depression, and other dysphoric moods.
   2. There are often features of borderline personality disorder, and in some cases both diagnoses may be warranted.
   3. Some of the individuals in this group would be considered eccentric because they are interested in fringe religious groups or are bigoted.

IX. Histrionic personality disorder

A. Definition
   1. This disorder is also called *hysterical personality.*
   2. Persons with *histrionic personality* disorder have a pattern of theatrical behavior that is overly reactive, intensely expressed, and perceived by others as shallow, superficial, or insincere; interpersonal relationships are characteristically disturbed; and their sexual adjustment is poor (*DSM*-III).
      a. Their behavior is often exhibitionistic, drawing attention to themselves by exaggerated expression of emotions ("playing a role").
      b. They inappropriately over-react to minor stimuli.
      c. Their interpersonal relationships are initially apt to be superficially warm, charming, and appealing; once a relationship is established, they become demanding and inconsiderate of others. They are often regarded as vain, egocentric, and self-absorbed.
      d. Despite outward displays of sexuality such as flirtatiousness and coquetry, these individuals are often naive and frigid.
      e. The disorder, when found in men, is often associated with the homosexual arousal pattern.

B. Case example

Scarlett O'Hara, the heroine of Margaret Mitchell's *Gone with the Wind,* seems to be a histrionic personality type. At the end of the novel, after she is rejected by Rhett Butler, she can't think of letting him go and thinks, "I won't think of it now—I'll go home to Tara tomorrow—I'll think of it all tomorrow at Tara. I can stand it then. Tomorrow, I'll think of some way to get him back. After all, tomorrow is another day."

X. Narcissistic personality disorder
A. Definition
The essential features are a grandiose sense of self-importance or uniqueness; preoccupation with fantasies of unlimited success; an exhibitionistic need for constant attention and admiration; characteristic responses to threats to self-esteem; characteristic disturbances in interpersonal relationships, such as lack of empathy, entitlement, interpersonal exploitiveness, and relationships that vacillate between the extremes of over-idealization and devaluation (*DSM*-III).
1. The exaggerated sense of self-importance may be manifested as extreme self-centeredness and self-absorption.
2. The fantasies are associated with unrealistic goals, involving unlimited ability, power, wealth, brilliance, beauty, or ideal love.
3. In seeking admiration and attention, narcissistic personalities are more concerned with appearances than with substance.
4. Their self-esteem is fragile.
5. Their interpersonal relationships are invariably disturbed by lack of empathy, feelings of entitlement, and taking advantage of others.
6. Their relationships tend to vacillate.
7. They usually exploit their relationships for their own gratification. In addition, they need constant flattery from others and usually maintain a gathering of people around them for such purposes.

B. Associated features
Histrionic, borderline, and antisocial personality characteristics are frequently found in association with this disorder.

C. Case example

J. C., a thirty-two-year-old corporate junior executive, was initially seen in consultation, jointly with his wife, because of marital distress. This was his second marriage and the couple had two children in elementary school. His wife complained that he was extremely self-centered and was always cool and distant with her. He was also remote from the children, but expected them to accomplish much to enhance his own name.

At work, he prided himself on his ruthless decisiveness in dealing with subordinates who might show signs of incompetency. About his superiors, he privately acknowledged that he would "play on their sympathy and compassionate feelings" to enhance his corporate position. He also confided that he had numerous brief extra-marital affairs, and on a few occasions had homosexual encounters. A handsome man, he prided himself on his sexual technique and his ability to be able to enjoy both sexes.

In discussing his work relationships, it became clear that he had no loyalty to any colleague or company policy and felt that he would leave to establish his own business to "run things my own way." He had had some strong disagreements with some of his superiors about his own practices, which were at odds with the ethics of the company.

It was believed that part of his own motivation for seeking joint consultation was that he felt a divorce would cost him more financially and hinder his business plans. He felt that he could reduce the financial cost by superficially complying with his wife's wishes.

He abruptly announced his plans to terminate the counseling, and did so.

XI. Antisocial personality disorder

A. Definition

1. Synonyms are *sociopathic personality disturbance; psychopathic personality; sociopath; psychopath; semantic disorder.*

2. The essential features are a history of continuous and chronic antisocial behavior in which the rights of others are violated; onset before age fifteen; the persistance of antisocial behavior after the age of fifteen into adult life; and failure to sustain good job performance over a period of several years. The same behavior pattern in a person younger than eighteen is diagnosed as a *conduct disorder* (*DSM*-III).

   a. Such persons are basically unsocialized and callous, and offer plausible rationalizations for their antisocial behavior.

   b. They tend to regard themselves as victims or to focus on minor or irrelevant aspects of antisocial incidents to detract from their accountability.

   c. They manifest their conflicts by acting out.

   d. Their behavior is chiefly antisocial, asocial, and amoral in character.

B. Prevalence

1. The exact incidence of antisocial personality disorder is not known, partly because of the lack of agreement among authorities about what kind of personality disturbance should be classified as antisocial.

2. Public mental hospitals have low admission rates for antisocial personalities. However, this probably does not reflect the actual incidence of the disorder, since many antisocial personalities are sent to prison for their offenses against society. In addition, most hospitals try to exclude antisocial persons because they are not equipped to deal with such patients.

3. Most people with antisocial personality are found in the lower socioeconomic groups, largely with backgrounds of rejection, deprivation, neglect, and abuse.

4. This disorder is much more common in males than females, and its onset tends to be earlier in males. *DSM*-III estimates prevalence in American men as about 3 percent and less than 1 percent in American women.
5. The fathers of those affected often have the same disorder.
C. Symptoms
   1. Behavior during childhood
      a. The onset of antisocial behavior occurs before the age of fifteen.
      b. Behavior is unsocialized and dominated by primitive drives.
      c. Emotional immaturity and impulsiveness are characteristic.
      d. Destructive, deceitful, obstinate, quarrelsome, and defiant behavior is frequent.
      e. Temper tantrums or outbursts of rage may occur.
      f. Delinquent behavior is found, such as truancy, theft, expulsion from school, running away from home, persistent lying, unusually early or aggressive sexual behavior, vandalism, chronic violations of rules at home or school, underachievement in school. (According to *DSM*-III, a history of two or more of these is one of the diagnostic criteria.)
      g. Enuresis is common.
   2. Behavior during adolescence (after the age of fifteen)
      a. Rebelliousness against parental or other forms of authority.
      b. Resistance to accepting the value system of the family.
      c. Conflict with school authorities and poor academic performance.
      d. Exaggeration of all these traits, as the person approaches adulthood, because of increased responsibility as well as the weakening of the restraining forces of family ties.
   3. Behavior in adult life
      a. Poor occupational performance for several years, as shown by frequent job changes, unemployment, absenteeism, or poor academic performance.
      b. Three or more arrests for offenses other than traffic violations or conviction for a felony.
      c. Two or more divorces or separations.
      d. Repeated physical fights or assaults.
      e. Repeated thefts, whether or not detected.

       f. Illegal occupations, such as selling drugs, pimping, or prostitution.

       g. Repeated defaulting on debts or other major financial responsibilities.

       h. Traveling from place to place without a prearranged job or clear goal for the period of travel or a clear idea of when the travel would terminate.

       i. Alcoholism and drug abuse are seen with increasing frequency.

  4. Generalization

  Not *all* the above behavior at the various life stages is found in each case.

D. Etiology

  1. The causes of antisocial personality disorder are not really known.

  2. Genetic

  Earlier reports stressed the "constitutional" aspects of the disorder. This emphasis grew out of the observations of those who noted the beginning of difficulty with parents in early years and a continuing difficulty in interpersonal relationships throughout life. Since the course seemed so inexorable, constitutionality was invoked as the chief etiological factor.

  3. Family history

  A history of antisocial personality disorder is often found in the fathers of both males and females with the disorder.

  4. Multiple causation

  Recent studies indicate that both genetic and environmental influences are important (*DSM*-III).

  5. Organic

  Some cases of antisocial behavior have been precipitated by brain damage, for example, by severe head trauma or encephalitis. Although the behavior may be classified as antisocial, technically such individuals are not usually considered antisocial personalities, but are more properly diagnosed as having organic mental disorders.

  6. Psychosocial

  Some authorities consider psychological and social factors to be chiefly responsible for the development of antisocial personality disorder.

    a. Social factors

      (1) The antisocial personality comes largely from the lower socioeconomic groups. There is a high rate of delinquency in the slum areas of larger urban communities.

          (2) Living according to the pleasure principle without regard for the reality principle is in part determined by social factors as well as by parental relationships.

          (3) The families and environment from which antisocial persons come have high rates of broken homes, alcoholism, and antisocial behavior.

  b. Psychological factors

    Johnson and Szurek describe the "superego lacunae" that developed in antisocial personalities as a result of unconscious fostering of such behavior by the parents during the developmental years.

E. Psychopathology

  1. The essential defect in antisocial personalities involves their character structure (hence, this disturbance is sometimes called a *character disorder* or *character neurosis*).

  2. Like infants, antisocial personalities give direct expression to their impulses. They are seemingly incapable of adapting their urges to the demands of society and unable to postpone immediate gratification of their desires.

  3. They defy, or come into conflict with, authority, and they lack sensitivity to other people's feelings.

  4. Since they are dominated by unsocialized drives, they have difficulty in their relationships with others. Although intellectually they recognize that their acts are illegal or unethical, they seem uninfluenced by such knowledge.

  5. They might be considered emotionally deficient. They are egocentric, selfish, make excessive demands, and are unable to view their own behavior objectively. They are usually free of anxiety, remorse, or guilt.

  6. From the foregoing, it becomes apparent that the antisocial person has a poorly developed conscience (defective superego).

    a. Conscience is largely dependent upon relationships with parents or parent substitutes. One's value system is usually developed through one's relationships with parents (largely by identification) and is based on affection and trust.

    b. In antisocial persons, the identification process is faulty. Either they are unable to evolve a value system through the normal process of identification or they develop pathological types of identification.

      (1) *Hostile identification* is internalization of undesirable personality traits of parents or authority figures.

      (2) *Identification with the aggressor* is internalization of the characteristics of a frustrated or feared parent or parent substitute.

    c. We often find a history of difficulty with parents or authority figures from the earliest years.

d. This history seems related to parental attitudes that are commonly unreasonable, neglectful, cruel, hypocritical, or inconsistent (i.e., vacillating or unpredictable). The child has difficulty attaching himself to either parent as an example to follow or as a source of security because there has been a lack of mutual affection, tenderness, or trust.

e. Because of this detachment from parents and parent-figures, the behavior of antisocial personalities develops no sense of direction (that is, they are uninfluenced by any concepts of right and wrong).

f. Some authorities feel that, in a sense, their willful, unsocialized behavior is a seeking for attention, affection, and acceptance.

F. Case report

Bob, the eighteen-year-old son of well-to-do parents, was brought to the hospital for psychiatric examination upon the order of a judge. One night four weeks earlier, the patient had, in the company of three other boys, entered a cemetery, tipped over several gravestones, and mutilated a monument.

When Bob first entered grade school, he had some minor difficulties. He performed below his intellectual capacity and frequently did things that the other children considered "daring" such as letting the air out of automobile tires. At nine, he began to smoke, not just experimentally, like some of the other boys, but often and somewhat defiantly.

He first came into difficulty with the law at the age of eleven when he stole two cigarette lighters and a wristwatch from a jewelry store. Following this, he was sent to a military boarding school upon the advice of the judge and the family physician. Two months after he entered the new school, he broke into the school store, stole candy and cigarettes, and ran away to a nearby city. He was found two days later in a hotel room by himself. He was returned to his home and completed the school year at the local school.

At thirteen, he and two other boys stole a large amount of gasoline from a nearby storage plant. This was used in a "jalopy" purchased for the patient by his father. At first, he denied the theft but, when confronted with irrefutable proof, admitted his guilt; however, he was unable to give any reason for wanting the gasoline. From the age of thirteen until seventeen, he was frequently involved in minor delinquencies but always escaped punishment because of his family's position in the community and because his father always made restitution. At seventeen, he began drinking beer and shortly was getting "high" regularly.

Bob was the older of two brothers but was reared as an only child because his infant brother died when Bob was four. After this, the parents overindulged him. At five, he fell from a horse, following which he had a few convulsions. He was examined at a well-known clinic and placed on anticonvulsants. After a few weeks of this treatment, he quit taking the medications. He says he has never been really close to anyone and has never felt toward his parents as other youngsters do.

Although the parents verbally disapproved of his behavior, they encouraged it in subtle ways; for example, increasing his already overly generous allowance after he was caught stealing from a hardware store.

At no time has he ever shown any guilt for his delinquent and antisocial behavior, and he always seems free of anxiety. His case illustrates some of the typical aspects of the antisocial personality disorder.

XII. Borderline personality disorder
  A. Definition

    The essential feature is instability in a variety of areas, including interpersonal relationships, behavior, mood, and self-image (*DSM-III*).

    1. Interpersonal relationships are often intense and unstable, with marked shifts of attitudes.

    2. Behavior is frequently impulsive, unpredictable, and potentially damaging.

    3. Mood is often unstable, shifting markedly from normal to dysphoric, and characterized by inappropriateness, intense anger, or lack of control of anger.

    4. Self-image may be profoundly disturbed, as manifested by uncertainty about several issues relating to identity, such as self-image, gender identity, and long-term goals or values.

  B. Previous labels for borderline personality disorder include *ambulatory schizophrenia, latent schizophrenia, pre-schizophrenia, schizophrenic character, abortive schizophrenia, pseudo-neurotic schizophrenia,* and so forth.

  C. The concept of borderline personality function has been developed largely through the ego-psychology school of psychoanalytic thinking.

  D. The borderline personality uses primitive psychotic-like defensive operations, such as denial, projection, splitting, and projective identification (see the chapter, "Adaptations to Anxiety").

  E. Masterson sees the borderline personality in adolescence as characterized by a persistent symbiosis with parental figures. There is a predominance of negative feelings that are shared by parent and child, which persists and yet binds the two together by mutual guilty and bad feelings.

  F. In summary, *borderline personality* is a term that applies to a level of disorganization. It is frequently associated with schizotypal, histrionic, or narcissistic personality. An example is the diagnosis, narcissistic personality with borderline features. The borderline state is a stable condition, not really a latent schizophrenia or pre-psychotic condition. The disorder appears to have most of its origin in dynamic and developmental aspects of childhood, rather than biochemical or hereditary factors. More specifically, families that use primitive and psychotic-like defensive operations tend to create an atmosphere to which their offspring adapt by similar defensive operations.

  G. Treatment
    1. Setting
      Patients usually respond to structure in both inpatient and outpatient settings, although the condition can be seen and diagnosed more clearly in a relatively unstructured setting.
    2. Medicine
      The response to antipsychotic medicine has not produced the results reported in the treatment of other psychotic disorders.
    3. Psychoanalytic therapy has been helpful.
    4. Some patients form relationships with their doctors that are virtually interminable.

XIII. Avoidant personality disorder
  A. Definition
    The essential features are hypersensitivity to rejection and unwillingness to enter into relationships unless given unusually strong guarantees of uncritical acceptance; social withdrawal, yet a desire for affection and acceptance; and low self-esteem (*DSM*-III).
    1. Unlike schizoid personalities, who are also socially isolated, individuals with avoidant personality disorder yearn for affection and acceptance.
    2. Avoidant disorder in childhood or adolescence is a predisposing factor.
  B. Prevalance
    The disorder is apparently more common among women.

XIV. Dependent personality disorder
  A. Definition
    The essential features are getting others to assume responsibility for major areas of one's life; subordinating one's own needs to those of others on whom one is dependent in order to avoid having to rely on oneself; lack of self-confidence; intense discomfort when alone for more than brief periods (*DSM*-III).
    1. The person abdicates all major decisions.
    2. The needs of the individuals upon whom the person is dependent dominate relationships.
    3. Such persons tend to belittle themselves and their abilities.
    4. They feel helpless when alone.
  B. Prevalence
    The disorder is diagnosed more frequently in women.

XV. Compulsive personality disorder
A. Definition

The essential features are a restricted ability to express warm and tender emotions; preoccupation with rules, order, organization, efficiency, and details, with a loss of ability to focus on "the big picture"; insistence that others submit to the person's way of doing things; excessive devotion to work and productivity to the exclusion of pleasure; and indecisiveness (*DSM*-III).

1. Such persons are stingy with their emotions.
2. They are conventional, serious, and lack charm and grace.
3. They are excessively preoccupied with trivial details, procedures, or forms.
4. They stubbornly insist that people submit to their way of doing things, although they are oppositional when subjected to the will of others.
5. Work and productivity are prized to the exclusion of pleasure and the value of interpersonal relationships.
6. Decision making is avoided, postponed, or protracted because of an inordinate fear of making a mistake.

B. Etiology
1. The person who possesses such traits is referred to as an *anancastic personality* or *anal character* (such an individual needs to feel in control of himself or herself and the environment).
2. According to psychoanalytic theory, such anal qualities develop in the infant during the period of toilet training (the anal phase of infantile sexuality).
3. According to learning theory, obsessions are conditioned responses to anxiety, and compulsions are behavioral patterns that reduce the anxiety.

C. Case example

A fifty-two-year-old financial officer of a large corporation consulted a psychiatrist because of his conflicts with his wife and his business associates. At the first interview, he stated that he was a very conscientious, inflexible, punctual, conforming man who had performed flawlessly within the corporation. However, the very traits which made his financial calculations so accurate also rendered him relatively inflexible in dealing with human beings. For example, he was very critical of his boss and his colleagues for being late to work or for any infraction of company policy or rules. He was critical of his wife's neatness, punctuality, and housework.

He planned to continue in treatment to help himself become more flexible.

XVI. Passive-aggressive personality disorder

    A. Definition

The essential feature is a resistance to demands for adequate activity or performance in both occupational and social functioning that is not expressed directly; as a consequence, there is pervasive and long-standing social or occupational ineffectiveness. The name of this disorder is based on the inference that such individuals are passively expressing covert hostility.

        1. Resistance means the person resents and opposes any demands either to increase or maintain a given level of functioning, made by others. This occurs most clearly at work. Resistance is not expressed directly, but rather through such maneuvers as procrastination, dawdling, stubbornness, intentional inefficiency, and "forgetfulness."

        2. As a result of the personality traits, the individual is ineffective both socially and occupationally.

    B. Case example

F. S., a thirty-four-year-old married man, was referred to the court's psychiatric consultant for evaluation after he had pleaded guilty to a charge of assault and battery and drunkenness upon a complaint filed by his wife, who reported that he came home drunk and threatened her with a knife. He had one previous arrest as a juvenile for malicious destruction of property and two prior arrests as an adult, one for drunkenness and the other for drunken driving.

During the interview, he blamed his drinking on his family troubles. He felt there had been a lot of pressures within his marriage for the preceding three or four years, and he particularly implicated his father-in-law as playing a prominent role in the conflict between him and his wife. He was critical of his wife and said that she was dominated by her mother and, although faithful, shiftless. He felt he was unable to communicate with either his father-in-law or his wife because they were both illiterate. Although he admitted that most of his complaints about his wife were minor, he felt they added up to incompatibility. He felt that his wife constantly aggravated him by her behavior and that this led to numerous arguments and difficulties. When not drinking, he was passive and not at all aggressive toward his wife. He had consulted numerous physicians for various physical problems, including hypoglycemia. He had been unemployed for the preceding year. There was no history of aggressive behavior toward other people nor had he ever been involved in altercations with men.

XVII. Treatment of personality disorders

    A. Treatment of the personality disorders is very difficult because the patients usually lack any fundamental motivation for change.

B. The positive rewards of their behavior overbalances the socially incurred ill-feeling that may result.
C. When they do seek treatment it is often likely to be—
    1. Because of anxiety developing secondarily in response to the social repercussions of their behavior.
    2. At the insistence of another person (a parent, spouse, or employer).
    3. Because of the slowly developing awareness of an unsatisfactory life-style.
D. Intensive psychoanalytically oriented psychotherapy is useful in narcissistic personality disorders and borderline personality disorders.
E. In individual therapy, the therapist may focus on the individual's maladaptive behavior rather than on a discussion of his inner life.
F. Such persons often need a different model with whom to identify and from whom to obtain reliable information about their emotional impact on others. In general, the therapist must remain flexible and be prepared to take an active role in the treatment process if necessary.
G. Group therapy has been of some value.

References

American Psychiatric Association. *Diagnostic and Statistical Manual of Mental Disorders.* 3d ed. Washington, D. C., 1978–1979.

Cleckley, H. *The Mask of Sanity.* 4th ed. St. Louis: C. V. Mobsy Company, 1964.

Eaton, M. T., Jr,; Peterson, M. H.; and David, J. A. *Psychiatry.* 3d ed. Flushing, N. Y.; Medical Examination Publishing Company, 1976, chap. 7.

Freedman, A. M.; Kaplan, H. I.; and Sadock, B. J. *Modern Synopsis of Comprehensive Textbook of Psychiatry,* Vol. 2. Baltimore: Williams & Wilkins Company, 1976, chap. 21.

Goodwin, D. W., and Guze, S. B. *Psychiatric Diagnosis.* New York: Oxford University Press. 2d ed. 1979, chap. 9.

Johnson, A. M., and Szurek, S. A. "The Genesis of Antisocial Acting Out in Children and Adults," *Psychoanalytic Quarterly* 21 (1952): 323–343.

Kernberg, O. *Borderline Conditions and Pathological Narcissism.* New York: Jason Aronson, 1975.

Kolb, L. C. *Modern Clinical Psychiatry.* 9th ed. Philadelphia: W. B. Saunders Company, 1977, chap. 24.

Masterson, J. *Treatment of the Borderline Adolescent: A Developmental Approach.* New York: Wiley-Interscience, 1972.

Nicholi, A. M., Jr., ed. *The Harvard Guide to Modern Psychiatry.* Cambridge: Belknap Press of Harvard University Press, 1978, chap. 14.

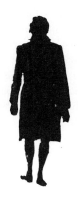

In order to do certain crazy things, it
is necessary to behave like a
coachman who has let go of the
reins and fallen asleep.

Jules Renard, *Journal,* **November,
1888.**

Disorders of
Impulse Control

I. Introduction

A. Not all antisocial behavior is identified with persons diagnosed as having *antisocial personality disorders.*

B. Excluded from the antisocial personality disorders are a group called neurotic characters, or acting-out neurotics, whose disturbance is characterized by the irresistible, repetitious expression of a *single* pleasurable impulse.

C. Antisocial behavior may be the expression of any type of impulse, but the specific symptom has a symbolic significance as related to the patient's life history.

D. In these disorders, the superego is usually well developed and is only defective to the extent that it permits acting out of one type of antisocial behavior.

E. In the past, these disorders were called impulse neuroses or impulse-ridden states. In the current nomenclature, they are called disorders of impulse control.

II. Definition

A disorder of impulse control is characterized by the following (*DSM*-III):

A. Failure to resist an impulse, drive, or temptation to perform some action that is harmful to the individual or to others. There may be conscious resistance to the impulse. The act may or may not be premeditated or planned.

B. Prior to committing the act, there is an increased sense of tension.

C. At the time of committing the act, there is an experience of either pleasure, gratification, or release. The act is ego-syntonic (acceptable to the ego). Immediately following the act, there may or may not be genuine regret, self-reproach, or guilt (*DSM*-III).

III. Specific categories

A. Pathological gambling

B. Kleptomania

C. Pyromania

D. Intermittent explosive disorder

E. Isolated explosive disorder

IV. Pathological gambling

A. Definition

The essential features of *pathological gambling* are a chronic and progressive preoccupation with gambling and the urge to gamble, and gambling behavior that compromises, disrupts, or damages personal, family and/or vocational pursuits. The gambling preoccupation, urge, and activity increase during periods of stress. Problems that arise as a result of the gambling lead to an intensification of the gambling behavior. These include loss of work due to absences in order to gamble, defaulting on debts and other financial respon-

sibilities, disrupted family relationships, borrowing money from illegal sources, forgery, fraud, embezzlement, and income tax evasion (*DSM*-III).
B. Associated features
The gambler usually appears overconfident, somewhat abrasive, very energetic, and is a free spender. When borrowing resources are strained, the likelihood of antisocial behavior occurs in order to obtain money for gambling. Any criminal behavior is typically non-violent, such as forgery, embezzlement, or fraud (*DSM*-III).
C. Case example

Mrs. J.P., the fifty-two-year-old wife of a social agency executive, was referred for psychiatric treatment because of her "addiction to bingo." Her gambling had its onset after she learned of the tragic death of her thirty-year-old scientist-son. Her irresistible urge to gamble (and lose) at bingo seemed to represent an equivalent of depression.

Repeated efforts at out-patient psychotherapy and hospital treatment were to little avail. She wrote worthless checks, stole, and went into debt to continue her habit. Ultimately, her husband divorced her. Unfortunately, there was no follow-up beyond that point.

V. Kleptomania
A. Definition
The essential feature of *kleptomania* is a recurrent failure to resist impulses to steal objects, not for immediate use or their monetary value. The objects taken are either given away, returned surreptitiously, or are kept hidden. Almost invariably, the individual has enough money to pay for the stolen objects. Prior to committing the act, there is an increasing sense of tension. At the time of committing the theft, there is an intense experience of gratification. Although the theft does not occur when immediate arrest is probable, it is not pre-planned and the chances of apprehension are not fully taken into account. Stealing is done without long-term planning and without assistance from, or collaboration with, others (*DSM*-III).
B. Sex-ratio
The majority of the individuals apprehended for shoplifting are female, but only a small portion of these have kleptomania.
C. Case example

A twenty-seven-year-old married man, who had just formed his own small business, consulted a psychiatrist about difficulties in his relationship with his wife and the hostile feelings he had toward his hypercritical father. He expressed a great deal of anger and negativism toward both parents, but especially toward the father, who was unreasonable, paranoid, and insensitive.

In discussing his past history, he reported that he had a habit of stealing small items from the shops he visited for business or personal reasons. These items were almost never of any use to him, and usually were inexpensive. He saved all of them and kept them in drawers in his workshop at home. No one knew of his stealing habit—not even his wife, who was irritated by what he described to her as his "impulse buying."

At first he reported no associated feelings with the stealing incidents, but later in therapy, he recalled that he felt anxious before and at the time of the thefts—and remorseful afterwards. He could not relate these incidents to any psychological determinant, but he suspected it had something to do with his rebellious feelings toward his father. He terminated therapy a few months later, when he left the city. At that time, he still did not know the reasons for his stealing.

(Note in the above: it was not the impulsive stealing that led to his seeking psychiatric treatment. The history of kleptomania was only incidentally reported in the therapeutic process.)

VI. Pyromania

A. Definition

The essential features of *pyromania* are recurrent failure to resist impulses to set fires and the intense fascination with the setting of fires and seeing fires burn. Prior to setting the fire, there is a buildup of tension. Once the fire is underway, the individual experiences intense pleasure or release. Although the fire-setting results from a failure to resist an impulse, there may be considerable advance preparation in order to get the fire underway (*DSM*-III).

B. Associated features

Alcohol intoxication, psychosexual dysfunction, lower then average I.Q., chronic personal frustration, and resentment toward authority figures in instances of pyromania. Cases have been described in which the individual was sexually aroused by a fire.

C. Case example

An eighteen-year-old married man was arrested for having set a number of fires in the city. In discussing the setting of the fires he indicated that he got a "thrill" or a "feeling of excitement" as he watched the fires. In addition, he experienced some sexual gratification from setting the fires. As a matter of fact, he would set the fires in an area in which he could witness them from his home and he and his wife would become sexually excited and have sexual intercourse while observing the blaze.

Apart from the particular offense that brought him to the attention of the law, there was evidence that he had had adjustment difficulties for many years. Obesity, for example, had been a problem with him for a long time, and he gave a history of an arrest four years earlier for an assault on a two-and-one-half-year-old boy. He felt that he turned to homosexuality at that point because he was not able to date in high school. He denied that he had had any homosexual feelings since he had been married in March of the previous year.

From clinical examination, there was no evidence that he was psychotic. In a general way, he indicated that he probably knew right from wrong and that at the time he set the first fire he knew it was wrong, but after that the rightness or wrongness of his behavior in setting additional fires did not enter his head—"It was just something I needed." There was also evidence that setting the fires relieved sexual, aggressive, and anxious feelings. At the time of the psychiatric examination in the county jail, he was still experiencing strong desires to set fires.

D. The pyromaniac must be distinguished from the arsonist.
VII. Intermittent explosive disorder
A. Definition
Intermittent explosive disorder is a new diagnostic category for individuals who have recurrent and paroxysmal episodes of significant loss of control of aggressive impulses that result in serious assault or destruction of property. The magnitude of the behavior during an episode is grossly out of proportion to any psychosocial stressors that may have played a role in eliciting the episodes or lack of control. The individual may describe the episodes as "spells" or "attacks." The symptoms appear within minutes or hours and, regardless of duration, remit almost as quickly. Following each episode, there is a genuine regret or self-reproach at the consequences of the action and the inability to control the aggressive impulses. Between the episodes, there are no signs of generalized impulsivity or aggressiveness. Previously, some of these individuals might have received a diagnosis of explosive personality (*DSM*-III).
B. Associated features
There may be prodromal affective or autonomic symptoms signaling an impending episode.
C. Case example

A twenty-two-year-old married man was referred to the psychiatric consultant to the court for evaluation after he had pleaded guilty to a charge of simple assault, growing out of an incident in which he was verbally and physically abusive to his wife. He was on probation at the time of the offense for a similar disorderly conduct offense committed nine months earlier.

At the interview, he was cooperative and pleasant but did not spontaneously volunteer much about himself. He was quiet, nonverbal, and not at all reflective. In discussing his difficulty he said, "Basically it's temper," which had been an issue in his marriage for the preceding three years. He said that the difficulty was that his temper began during the time that he was in the service for two years following his eighteenth birthday. "It just seemed to come on by itself." It had its onset shortly before he was sent overseas to Vietnam where he served as an infantry rifleman and was wounded.

The kind of subsequent anger that included the physical and verbal abuse of his wife occurred about every six months. At such times he usually would awaken angry and, as a consequence, would overreact throughout the entire day.

Mental status evaluation revealed him to be free of anxiety and depression. He didn't think that there was anything wrong with his mind and he denied delusions, hallucinations, and other types of perceptual distortions. He denied any thinking disturbance. He thought that it was sometimes hard for him to trust others.

It was the consultant's opinion that this man had an explosive personality. Since the outbursts seemed to develop in relationships chiefly with his wife, it was suggested that they both be referred for marriage counseling if the wife planned to remain in the marriage.

VIII. Isolated explosive disorder
  A. Definition

  This is a new diagnostic category for indiviudals who have had a *single* discrete episode, characterized by failure to resist an impulse that led to a single violent, externally directed act, which had a catastrophic impact on others, and for which the available information does not justify the diagnosis of schizophrenia, antisocial personality disorder, or conduct disorder. Previously called "catathymic crisis." *Isolated explosive disorder* is an unexpected, explosive outburst of impulsive, often destructive, behavior, understandable only in terms of unconscious motivation (*DSM*-III).

References

American Psychiatric Association. *Diagnostic and Statistical Manual of Mental Disorders.* 3d ed. Washington, D.C., 1978-1979.

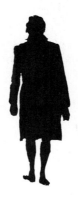

Love's mysteries in souls do grow,
But yet the body is his book.

John Donne: "The Ecstacy," in
Songs and Sonnets **(1633)**

Psychosexual Disorders

I. Definition

In the *Diagnostic and Statistical Manual of Mental Disorders,* 3d ed. (*DSM*-III), the psychosexual disorders are divided into four groups:

A. The gender identity disorders

Gender identity disorders are characterized by an individual's feeling of discomfort and inappropriateness about his or her anatomic sex and by persistent behavior generally associated with the other sex.

B. The paraphilias

The paraphilias are characterized by sexual arousal in response to objects or situations that are not normally arousing and by gross impairment of the capacity for affectionate sexual activity with human partners.

C. The psychosexual dysfunctions

Psychosexual dysfunctions are inhibitions of the appetitive or psychophysiological changes that characterize the sexual response cycle.

D. Other psychosexual disorders include the disorder ego-dystonic homosexuality, covered here as a gender identity disorder.

II. Introductory comments

A. Sexual deviations have been practiced throughout history and by all races.

B. Some deviant acts may be considered to be within the normal range of sexual expression if indulged in only sporadically or as foreplay to normal coitus.

C. Sexual deviancy includes any sexual behavior that is at variance with more-or-less culturally accepted norms.

D. To be considered deviant, either the quality or the object of the sexual drive must be deemed abnormal.

E. Our concepts of sexual normalcy and deviancy are related to the values of our society. Since these values change, concepts and definitions of sexual deviance also change.

F. Some authorities speak of "sexual variants" rather than "sexual deviancies."

G. This group of disorders contains those that were classed as sexual deviations in *DSM*-II (i.e., the paraphilias), plus psychosexual dysfunctions which were classified as psychophysiologic disorders in *DSM*-II.

H. Although we classify the gender disorders and paraphilias as distinct entities, they frequently overlap.

I. The deviant is usually one who has difficulty achieving normal or satisfactory sexual relations with a mature human partner. Thus, according to Marmor, the deviant practices represent alternative ways of attempting to achieve sexual gratification.

III. Classification
A. Gender identity disorders

In this chapter, the following are considered to be gender identity disorders.
1. Transsexualism
2. Homosexuality (In *DSM*-III, this is classified under Other Psychosexual Disorders as "ego-dystonic homosexuality.")

B. Paraphilias
1. Fetishism (found almost exclusively in males)
2. Transvestism
3. Zoophilia
4. Pedophilia
5. Exhibitionism
6. Voyeurism
7. Sexual masochism
8. Sexual sadism
9. Sadomasochism
10. Atypical paraphilias

C. Psychosexual dysfunctions

IV. Transsexualism
A. Definition

The essential features are a persistent sense of discomfort and inappropriateness about one's anatomic sex and a persistent wish to be rid of one's genitals and to live as a member of the opposite sex (*DSM*-III). Such persons frequently choose to wear the clothing and to engage in activities that are considered characteristic of the opposite sex.

B. Types

Three major types are listed in *DSM*-III: (1) "asexual," the person who denies ever having strong sexual feelings; (2) "homosexual"; and (3) "heterosexual," the individual who claims to have had an active heterosexual life.

C. Course

Chronic, and unremitting without treatment

D. Treatment
1. Psychiatric treatment of this disorder has been disappointing.
2. Psychotherapy has been unsuccessful.
3. Aversive therapy has also been unsuccessful.
4. Sex transformation, or reconstructive surgery, has been used for a carefully screened group of patients. Persons with psychotic or borderline behavior, a criminal record, or gross sexual disturbances have been excluded. Although such surgery does not always relieve symptoms (e.g., depression), the patients seem to have done well post-operatively. Some authorities state that in the absence of long-term follow-up studies, the outcome remains controversial.

E. Case example

A twenty-four-year-old, single genetic male was admitted to the hospital for transsexual surgery. He had been born in a small town in southern Minnesota and had an unusually healthy life.

He stated that from his earliest memories he had regarded himself as a girl and that throughout his life he had never felt differently. Some of his earliest memories were of dressing up in the clothes of his sister, who was two years older. He was interested exclusively in dolls, little girls' games, and playing with girls. He did not like playing with boys or engaging in their games. He was also interested in dolls and cooking and, in high school, baton twirling. He said that he was always accepted "as a girl" by the girls in the small town in which he grew up.

By the end of grade school, he was taunted by boys for his feminine ways. It was during his midteens, while coming across descriptions of a famous case of transsexuality, that it began to dawn upon him that he might be a transsexual.

He denied any overt sexual experiences of any type except for a few anal sexual experiences. He was afraid of having relationships with a male "because he would quickly find out about me." He had never attempted sexual relations with a genetic female— "this would disgust me." He masturbated frequently and in his fantasies played the role of a woman, lying on his back and accepting the penis from his imaginary male lover.

About four and one-half years earlier, he had begun to take estrogens and dress and live like a woman. During this time, there was substantial breast development, his male genitalia became "smaller," and he became unable to have erections. He felt disgust for his penis and testicles, never felt them, and kept them constantly tucked between his legs. He also enrolled in a school for beauticians, where he met his first fellow transsexual. About two years before admission to the hospital, he had his breasts injected with liquid silicone to make them "more solid."

He was a natural blond and had never had much trouble with excessive bodily and facial hair. He had a "peaches-and-cream" complexion, and a depilatory used about every ten days controlled the relatively small amount of facial fuzz. In the hospital, a one-stage transsexual operation was performed.[1]

V. Homosexuality

A. In the new classification (*DSM*-III) homosexuality *per se* is not classified as a deviancy. Although the American Psychiatric Association has officially taken the position that homosexuality does not constitute a psychiatric disorder, the issue remains controversial. Some clinicians believe that homosexuality should always be considered deviant; others claim that there is inadequate scientific evidence that homosexuality is based on unconscious conflicts.

1. Courtesy of the late Donald W. Hastings, M. D., University of Minnesota Hospitals.

B. In *DSM*-III, ego-dystonic homosexuality is listed. This category is for individuals whose sexual interests are directed primarily toward people of the same sex *and* who are either disturbed by, in conflict with, or wish to change their sexual orientation.

C. Prevalence
   1. According to Kinsey, about 4 percent of white males consider themselves homosexuals.
   2. Homosexuals are of all socioeconomic classes.
   3. Homosexuals tend to be attracted to urban areas and to beaches known to have substantial homosexual communities.

D. Types of homosexuals
   1. Many homosexuals openly live the "gay" or Lesbian life. A diminishing number live as heterosexuals. These bisexuals frequently marry and have families. They carry out their homosexual lives in secret and relatively infrequently.
   2. Although the statement is becoming less true, certain occupations still tend to attract homosexuals. Among them are competitive sports, military groups, interior decorating, dancing, and hairdressing.

E. Etiology
   1. Constitutional factors
      a. There are heterosexual and homosexual components of the libidinal drives of everyone. Our sexual behavior is related to our sexual identification and, also, to our ability to sublimate certain drives.
      b. A surfacing of homosexual drives has been attributed by some to genetic or biologic factors.
   2. Psychoanalytic theory
      a. According to this theory, castration anxiety and unresolved oedipal situations underlie male homosexuality.
      b. The male homosexual has identified with his mother.
      c. The female homosexual has identified with her father.
   3. Environmental theories
      a. Some authorities believe that homosexual men have overly close, intimate, possessive, dominating, overprotective, and "demasculinizing" mothers, and detached, unaffectionate, hostile fathers who treat their sons in a humiliating way.
      b. Similarly, homosexual females are said to have submissive fathers who were distant to their daughters, and mothers who were hostile, competitive, defeminizing, and who favored sons.
      c. Seduction in early life by a homosexual may, in rare cases, play a significant etiological role.

4. Cultural theories
   a. Homosexuality has existed in both past and present cultures. It has often been viewed as a normal variant of biological behavior. However, there are cultures in which homosexuality is unknown.
   b. Subcultures in which there is an undue restriction on any show of heterosexual interest (e.g., prohibition of dating, dancing, and so forth) may lead to the belief that homosexual behavior is less forbidden than heterosexual behavior.
   c. Homosexuality may occur transiently—in adolescents, as an expression of curiosity or experimentation, or in circumstances where heterosexual contacts are unavailable (e.g., American prisons).

F. Clinical types
   1. Some clinicians still refer to two types of homosexuality:
      a. Latent homosexuality
         When homosexuality is *latent,* the homosexual desires are largely unconscious, unrecognized, and projected or sublimated. Latency varies inversely with the strength of repression.
      b. Overt homosexuality
         Homosexuality is considered *overt* when it is consciously recognized. This recognition may or may not affect the person's appearance.
         (1) Most homosexuals are normal in appearance.
         (2) Some show some of the outward behavioral characteristics of the opposite sex. For example, some male homosexuals are effeminate in appearance and manner and some homosexual women seem masculine.

G. Treatment
   1. Of the basic underlying homosexuality
      a. Most homosexuals do not seek treatment. It is only those who seek surgery or who have incidental psychological symptoms or personality problems that do.
      b. Psychoanalysis
         Intensive psychotherapy has been reported as having favorable results in a significant number who sought treatment and wanted change.
      c. Behavioral modification
         Negative conditioning, in which the showing of homoerotic pictures has been accompanied by injection of apomorphone (to produce vomiting) or painful electrical stimuli, has had some reported success.

       d. Drug therapy
         (1) Tranquilizers or antidepressants have been pre-scribed for coincidental anxiety or depression.
         (2) Male hormones seem contraindicated for homosexual males since they only increase the sexual drive without changing the aim.
       e. Group therapy has been said to have beneficial results.
       f. Some therapists approach the treatment of homosexuality as if it represents inhibition of sexual desire (inhibited appetitive phase type of psychosexual dysfunction)
    2. Of incidental emotional symptoms or personality problems
      In general, treatment follows the same rules that apply to heterosexual people with these problems.
H. Case example

A twenty-seven-year-old single man consulted a psychiatrist after he had been rejected for induction into the army. He said that as far back as the age of ten, he had been troubled with strong homosexual urges. On one occasion in the tenth grade, he developed such a strong attraction for another boy that he became "very ill" for several days and had to remain home in bed.

After graduating from art school, he obtained employment as a commercial artist and had remained successfully employed in that capacity. He had a few casual acquaintances but almost no close friends. Because of his homosexual desires, he purposely avoided forming friendships with other men.

His father was described as a gentle, mild-mannered man. His mother was described as quite the opposite—stern, "unfeminine," and "hot-tempered." She administered the discipline in the family and, though she assumed a rather masculine role, was usually sick in bed one or two days every two weeks. The patient was closer to his mother than to his father.

The patient had been able to control his homosexual desires until about two years earlier when, under the influence of alcohol, he allowed another man to seduce him. Since that time he had had a few homosexual experiences. Because of his great guilt, he has made strenuous efforts to control his urges.

VI. Fetishism
  A. Definition
    1. The essential features are the use of inanimate objects as the preferred or exclusive method of producing sexual excitement. The inanimate love object is often associated with the body; for example, underwear or stockings.
    2. Preoccupation with certain parts of the female body (e.g., breasts, buttocks, legs, hips) is called *partialism*.
    3. The fetish is used as the masturbatory object, thus it is clearly a symbolic substitute for the female, rather than the male, genital.

B. Prevalence
  1. Fetishism seems to be peculiar to men.
  2. Kinsey believed that there was a relationship between sado-masochistic behavior and fetishism.
  3. No figures are available on its prevalence.
  4. Sometimes a fetishist is arrested for stealing an article of female clothing, especially undergarments ("fetish theft").
C. Etiology
  1. Freud attributed fetishism to the castration anxiety originating in early childhood.
     a. The fetish represents a symbolic "female penis" and reassures the male that the female also has a penis, thus allaying castration anxiety.
     b. Such theories are of dubious value since castration anxiety is seen as a cause of many disorders that are not sexual deviations.
  2. Like many homosexuals, fetishists do not achieve a healthy identification with their fathers who, according to Marmor, have usually been distant, absent, or rejecting.
D. Treatment
  1. As in other sexual deviations, motivation to change is critical.
  2. Psychotherapy is focused on the patient's basic feelings of masculine inadequacy and heterosexual inhibition.
  3. Group psychotherapy may be helpful.
  4. Behavioral therapy has been tried.
  5. Marmor believes that a combination of dynamic and behavioral techniques may ultimately prove the most effective therapy.
E. Case example

A twenty-eight-year-old married man was referred to the court's psychiatric consultant after he had been arrested for touching an eighteen-year-old girl on the buttocks on two occasions on a downtown street. He admitted that he had touched between thirty to fifty girls usually between fourteen and twenty-one-years old, on the buttocks, breasts, or genitalia. He rarely touched the same girl twice. In addition, he admitted that on three or four occasions he had made obscene propositions to the girls. He said the incidents usually occurred on his way to work or on his way home in the evening and were most apt to occur when his wife was menstruating and unavailable for sexual relationships. In all instances he denied having an erection or an orgasm, but he did describe a feeling of "excitement" that he compared to the experience he had in other situations, such as shooting deer. He denied other kinds of sexual problems, claiming that he got along well with his wife.

During the interview, he behaved very much like a schizoid person, showing a rather blunted affect and a lack of verbal spontaneity. He said that on many occasions in the past he had vowed to himself to give up his deviancy but had always found it difficult to stop.

He was recommended for probationary supervision with the stipulation that he attend a psychiatric clinic.

VII. Transvestitism
A. Definition

The essential feature is sexual arousal from wearing the clothes of the opposite sex. The behavior is recurrent and persistent, and interference with it results in intense frustration.

B. Prevalence
1. Children sometimes dress up in the garb of the opposite sex.
2. Tranvestitism is more frequently found in males. In our culture, dressing in the clothes of the opposite sex is considered less deviant in females.
3. Some authorities say transvestitism is frequently associated with other deviations, and some describe a triad of deviancy characterized by transvestitism, fetishism, and homosexuality.

C. Etiology

In addition to what has been said previously about the etiology of sexual deviancy,
1. The confusion about sexual identification may date from the earliest years in the lives of such individuals.
2. The parents may have preferred a child of the opposite sex.
3. There may have been envy of the opposite sex role.
4. It is thought that the male transvestite reacts to his castration anxiety by identifying with the phallic woman. The mother of such patients is often reported as being seductive.
5. The female transvestite is regarded as having penis envy.

D. Prognosis

The prognosis is questionable; transvestites are reluctant to surrender their deviancy because the syndrome is pleasurable (ego-syntonic). Motivation for change usually results from external pressures.

E. Treatment

Because of the reluctance of transvestites to alter their behavior, treatment has been discouraging. In recent years there have been attempts at aversive behavioral therapy, using electroshocks or emetics.

F. Case example

R. U., a twenty-one-year-old married man, was referred to the court's psychiatric consultant after he had pleaded guilty to a disorderly conduct charge growing out of his arrest in a fitting room of the dress department of a department store, dressed in women's clothing.

Upon examination by the police physician, it was discovered that he was completely dressed in women's clothing, including a padded brassiere and women's hose. He admitted that he had dressed in women's clothing on a previous occasion, about two weeks earlier. He felt his problem was a climax to a rather deep-seated sexual problem and reported that he received a thrill upon entering the women's fitting room in the department store, as he had, previously, when he entered the women's washroom of a downtown theatre. Just wearing the clothing stimulated him sexually. He seemed to be immature and naive but did not show other evidences of sociopathic behavior. He was placed under probationary supervision and referred to a psychiatric clinic.

VIII. Zoophilia
A. Definition
   1. The essential feature is the use of animals as the preferred or exclusive method of producing sexual excitement. The animal may be the object of intercourse, or may be trained to sexually excite the human partner by licking or rubbing (*DSM*-III).
   2. Also called *bestiality*.
B. Prevalence
   1. Zoophilia is most commonly found in adolescents and usually involves a household pet or farm animal.
   2. Said to be more common in people who live in rural areas or are socially isolated.
   3. The disorder is apparently rare in other circumstances.
   4. Such patients are often schizoid, mentally retarded, or psychotic.
C. Case example
   In the following clinical vignette, the patient does not satisfy the current true criteria for zoophilia but does indicate zoophilic interests.

   Mrs. J. W., a thirty-year-old, married woman, came for psychiatric treatment because of depressive symptoms. These were in part a result of a somewhat estranged relationship with her husband who, although attentive, was not sexually interested in her. During the course of her hospitalization, she became profoundly depressed when her pet dog died. At that point she revealed that on a number of occasions she had engaged in sexual relations with the dog.

IX. Pedophilia
A. Definition
   The essential feature is the preference for repetitive sexual activity with prepubertal children of either sex.

B. Prevalence
1. Prevalence is most difficult to estimate, although it is most common in adult males.
2. Heterosexual offenses are more common than homosexual ones. The popular belief that homosexuals tend to be child molesters seems to be a myth.
3. Mostly, the behavior is genital petting. Most pedophiles do not resort to force or aggression.
C. Etiology
1. Most pedophiles are mild-mannered men who have profound feelings of masculine inadequacy and a fear of being castrated by mature women. They are frequently sexually impotent.
2. On the other hand, the male pedophile is often said to be masochistic.
3. Many of the men feel that their penis is small, hence children are seen as less threatening or less challenging.
4. Although no single family constellation is identifiable, a large percentage of pedophiles seem to come from unhappy home situations and to have had a poor relationship with the father.
D. Clinical types
Men who approach children sexually can be divided into the following groups:
1. Occasionally, males who are under the influence of alcohol
2. Males who are responding to a special situation
3. Pedophiles
4. Mentally retarded persons
5. Sociopathic types
6. Disorganized schizophrenics
7. Men with organic brain disease (senile dementia).
E. Case example

Mr. I. H., a thirty-six-year-old single man, was referred to the court's psychiatric consultant after he had pleaded guilty to drunkenness when he was found picking up a three-year-old boy and walking away with him. History revealed that he had been arrested on several occasions and had appeared in court three times. Seven years earlier, he had been picked up by police for questioning after there had been complaints in a neighborhood about his frequent appearances there when there were small children around. He was released. About five years earlier, he had been arrested for drunkenness and held in jail overnight. A few months later, he was arrested for disturbing the peace. On that occasion, he had picked up a three-year-old boy but claimed that he did nothing to him. About four years earlier, he was arrested on a charge of indecent assault after picking up a four-year-old girl. He said that he was so drunk at the time that he could not remember exactly what happened.

During the interview, he was quiet but frank in discussing his problem and his previous court appearances. There were certain schizoid qualities to his behavior. Although he admitted that he had a problem, he was not certain it was sexual. He felt that his basic attraction to children was toward those who were in need of care or attention. Mental-status examination did not reveal any signs of a disturbance in thinking or perception. He was committed to a state hospital under the sexual psychopathic law.

X. Exhibitionism

A. Definition

The essential feature is repetitively exposing the genitals to an unsuspecting stranger for the purpose of producing sexual excitement. The act of exposure constitutes the final sexual gratification. The term is sometimes used in the popular sense to describe somebody who is "showing off."

B. Prevalence

1. Exhibitionistic play among children is common and is not considered a deviancy.
2. It is one of the more common deviations among adults.
3. It is nearly always a deviation of males. Females usually do not derive erotic satisfaction from exhibiting their genitalia, but derive more pleasure from displaying other parts of their bodies.
4. The exhibitionist often returns repeatedly to the same scene to expose himself. As a consequence, he is frequently arrested.
5. In senile men, it may be a symptom of impaired judgment and poor impulse control.

C. Etiology

1. Psychodynamically, the exhibitionist seems to be seeking reassurance for his underlying castration anxiety.
2. The exposure may thus be an attempt to seek reassurance by
   a. Having another person react to the sight of his genitalia.
   b. Having other persons show fear of him.
   c. Showing the female what he wishes she could show him, thus reassuring himself that she also has a penis.
3. Some say that exhibitionists suffer from sexual impotence or premature ejaculation and deep-seated feelings of masculine inadequacy.

D. Prognosis

1. The prognosis depends upon the exhibitionist's desire for change.
2. It is also related to the severity of the deviancy.
3. The deviancy usually ceases with aging.

E. Treatment
1. The exhibitionist rarely seeks help voluntarily.
2. Treatment should be directed toward his underlying feelings of masculine inadequacy.
F. Case example

G. J., a thirty-six-year-old married man, was referred to the court's psychiatric consultant for evaluation after he had pleaded guilty to a charge of exposing himself to a woman in the downtown area. His history indicated that he had begun exposing himself several months earlier and, although he could not give any conscious reason for the behavior, it was interesting to note that he had become impotent shortly before he experienced the first urge to expose himself.

Although he indicated that he was worried about his impotence, he had not yet summoned up enough courage to discuss the matter with his personal physician. He seemed to have no understanding that his impotence might be psychogenic and that this might have some relationship to his exhibitionism. Mental-status examination did not reveal any thinking disorder or any major personality disturbance.

XI. Voyeurism
A. Definition
The essential feature is repetitive seeking out of situations in which the individual engages in looking at unsuspecting women who are either naked, in the act of disrobing, or engaging in sexual activity. The act of looking is accompanied by sexual excitement, frequently by orgasm accomplished by masturbation ("Peeping Tom").
B. Prevalence
1. Sexual curiosity is universal, and voyeuristic tendencies are widespread in the male population, as indicated by the extent to which nude or nearly nude women are used in the various communications media.
2. It is normal to be excited by the sight of a love object.
3. It is probably a common deviancy, although the extent is not known because voyeurs are quiet and unobtrusive and, hence, rarely caught.
C. Etiology
1. Voyeuristic urges are universal; it is the inability to keep them within socially accepted limits that poses problems.
2. The psychoanalytic explanation is centered on feelings of castration anxiety; the deviation provides reassurance.
3. Some authorities view this deviation as an attempt to recreate exciting and pleasurable childhood experiences with the mother.
D. Prognosis
1. Depends upon the voyeur's desire for change.
2. Is also related to the severity of the deviancy.

E. Treatment
   1. The voyeur rarely seeks help voluntarily.
   2. Treatment is an attempt to help the person deal with underlying feelings of inadequacy.
   3. Some patients say they suffer from impotence and premature ejaculation.
F. Case example

A twenty-three-year-old married man was examined by the court's psychiatric consultant after he had pleaded guilty to a charge of window-peeping.

He stated that he began his voyeuristic activities in his first year of college. He estimated that he peeped in windows about once every three or four months. In that period of time he had been picked up by the police on two occasions, but formally charged only once. He was a mild-mannered, frank, and open individual who was basically shy and retiring but could verbalize easily about his problem. He denied any other types of sexually deviant behavior and denied that he had ever been aggressive in any sexual or asocial way. He came from an upper-middle-class family and had an austere father who was emotionally remote from him. He described his mother as a seductive person who had never allowed him to have a warm relationship with his father.

Arrangements were made for him to be seen in a psychiatric clinic.

XII. Sexual masochism
A. Definition
   The essential feature is sexual excitement produced in an individual by his own suffering. As defined in *DSM*-III, the diagnosis is warranted under either of the first two following conditions:
   1. There has been intentional participation in an activity in which the individual was harmed or the individual's life was threatened in order to produce sexual excitement, which did occur.
   2. When the preferred or exclusive mode of producing sexual excitement is to be humiliated, bound, beaten, or otherwise made to suffer.
   3. *Flagellation* (erotic whipping) is one example of masochism.
   4. *Moral masochism* is the seeking of humiliation and failure rather than physical pain.
B. Prevalence
   1. Elements of mild masochism are common.
   2. The actual prevalence of this disorder is not known.
C. Etiology
   Again, castration anxiety is the psychoanalytic explanation for both moral and physical masochism.

D. Treatment
1. Treatment should be aimed at the underlying feelings of inadequacy.
2. Aversive therapies have been tried.
3. Perhaps a combination of dynamic psychotherapy and some behavioral therapy would offer the best prospect for resolution.

XIII. Sexual sadism
A. Definition
The essential feature is inflicting physical or psychological suffering on another person as a method of stimulating sexual excitement and orgasm, during which there are insistent and persistent fantasies in which sexual excitement is produced as a result of suffering inflicted on the partner. As defined in *DSM*-III, the diagnosis is warranted under the following three conditions:
1. The individual has repeatedly intentionally inflicted psychological or physical suffering on a nonconsenting partner in order to produce sexual excitement.
2. The preferred or exclusive mode of sexual excitement combines humiliation of a consenting partner with simulated or mildly injurious bodily suffering.
3. As in (2) above, but bodily injury is extensive, permanent, and possibly mortal.
4. Rape is an extreme form of sadism.
B. Prevalence
1. Mildly sadistic trends are common in all males.
2. The exact prevalence is not known.
3. Sadism also refers to other acts of excessive cruelty not related to sexuality, such as beating of children.
4. Extreme sadism is usually a psychotic symptom.
C. Etiology
According to psychoanalytic theory, underlying castration is the cause of this type of behavior, also.
D. Case example
Mr. Creakle, the cruel headmaster of Salemn House in *David Copperfield:*

"He [Creakle] then showed me the cane, and asked me what I thought of *that,* for a tooth? Was it a sharp tooth, hey? Was it a double tooth, hey? Had it a deep prong, hey? Did it bite, hey? At every question, he gave me a fleshy cut with it that made me writhe: so I was very soon made free of Salemn House—and was very soon in tears also."

XIV. Sado-masochism
A. Definition
1. The occurrence of sadism and masochism in the same person. These two deviancies often occur together, and Freud regarded masochism as sadism turned inward.
2. The two conditions are sometimes included under the term *algolagnia*. Thus, *active algolagnia* is sadism, and *passive algolagnia* is masochism.
B. Case example

A thirty-seven-year-old man, separated from his wife, was referred for psychiatric consultation by the attorney who was defending him in a suit filed by a woman who accused him of tying her up and beating her.

He reported that he had been aware of sado-masochistic feelings from about the age of eighteen, although he recalled pleasurable responses to being tied up by another boy at the age of eleven, when they played cowboy and Indian. Since his marriage at twenty-one, he had gone out with a number of women. He would derive sexual pleasure from either tying up a woman or being tied up by her. He usually terminated the relationship with sexual intercourse. He said he found that women liked to be treated roughly. For the preceding five years, he had intermittent sexual impotence.

XV. Other paraphilias
A. Incest
1. Definition
Sexual relations between members of the same family (e.g., parent-child, brother-sister).
2. Prevalence
a. The prevalence is unknown.
b. Although psychiatrists are aware that *incestuous feelings* are commonplace in their patients, they are also aware that most people erect strong defenses against them and that the incest taboo is a very powerful prohibition in most cultures.
3. Case example

A twenty-year-old college student was referred for psychiatric evaluation by a clergyman because he was sexually interested in his two teenage sisters, one of whom he had impregnated. He was a tense, anxious, nonverbal man who bit his fingernails. He described a difficult relationship with his father. Although he had intense sexual feelings toward his two sisters, he was "scared to death" when he dated other girls.

B. Excretory perversions
   Excretory perversions are of several types.
   1. *Coprophilia* is a pathological sexual interest in excretions. It includes the desire to defecate on a partner or to be defecated upon.
   2. *Coprophagia* is a desire to eat feces.
   3. *Coprolalia* is the compulsive utterance of obscene words.
   4. *Uralagnia* is the desire to urinate on a partner or to be urinated upon.
C. Frottage
   1. Definition of *frottage*
      Sexual pleasure is derived from rubbing or pressing against fully clothed members of the opposite sex. An individual so afflicted is called a frotteur, and the deviance is also known as *frotteurism.*
   2. Prevalence
      Usually a male deviation.
D. *Necrophilia* is the deriving of sexual gratification from corpses.
E. Telephone scatologia
   1. *Telephone scalologia* is sexual gratification derived, usually by men who telephone women, make obscene remarks, and suggest that the woman would meet them and engage in sexual activity. Also called *lewdness.*
   2. The man is usually apprehended when the woman agrees to meet him where the police can arrest him.
   3. Case example

      E. L., a twenty-year-old single male, was referred to the court's psychiatric consultant for evaluation after he had been arrested for making obscene phone calls to a sixteen-year-old girl over a six-month period. He would make such comments as, "Do you still have your cherry?" Or, "I want to put my fingers in your hairy cunt." Or, "If you don't let me fuck you, I will force you to fuck me." He admitted that he became sexually excited and on a couple of occasions masturbated when he made these phone calls.
      During the interview, he seemed uneasy and defensive and was not very revealing of himself. There was a certain strangeness about his behavior. He was evasive when questioned about his thought processes, although he denied any psychotic mentation, delusions, hallucinations, or other types of perceptual distortions. The MMPI profile suggested depression, passive dependency, and homosexual impulses.
      He was recommended for probationary supervision, with the stipulation that he be seen for further evaluation at the local mental health center to see if he could participate in any meaningful kind of treatment.

F. *Pyromania* is discussed in "Disorders of Impulse Control."

XVI. Prognosis for paraphiliacs

A. In general, the prognosis for paraphiliacs depends upon the severity and the chronicity of the deviation. When the paraphilia is well-developed and firmly fixed, and there is lack of desire for change, the prognosis is extremely poor.

B. The best prognosis seems to exist when there is a relationship between the deviant behavior and some precipitating environmental stress, and for younger deviants (especially adolescents).

C. Since the symptom is pleasurable (ego-syntonic), it is often difficult to treat, especially since deviants seldom seek psychiatric treatment on their own.

XVII. Treatment of paraphiliacs

A. There is no ideal treatment.

B. Psychotherapy is a long, drawn-out, and tedious process with sometimes doubtful results. For those who are uncomfortable, anxious, or depressed, an indication that they cannot accept their deviance, psychotherapy is more promising. Such treatment is usually psychoanalytically oriented.

C. Behavioral therapy has been tried with some reported success.

D. When the deviance is not well fixed, the patient is more likely to respond to either of the above therapies.

E. Group therapy has shown some promise.

F. Environmental manipulation is sometimes of value.

G. Sometimes confinement of the deviant is necessary for the protection of the community (e.g., the pedophile who repeatedly approaches young children).

XVIII. Psychosexual dysfunctions

A. Definition

1. The essential feature is inhibition of the appetitive or psychophysiological changes which characterize the complete sexual response cycle. Ordinarily, the diagnosis is only made when the disturbance is a major part of the presenting problem. It is not made if the sexual dysfunction is attributable to organic factors (*DSM*-III).

2. The sexual response cycle can be divided into the following phases (*DSM*-III):

a. Appetitive

The *appetitive phase* consists of sexual fantasies and sexual desire.

b. Excitement

Excitement is the subjective sense of sexual pleasure with accompanying physiological changes (penile tumescence and erection in the male; generalized pelvic vasocongestion with vaginal lubrication and swelling of the external genitalia in the female; and accompanying physiological changes).

    c. Orgasm

       Orgasm is the peaking of sexual pleasure accompanied by rhythmic contraction of the perineal muscles and pelvic reproductive organs and release of sexual tension (about 15 percent of women can only have clitoral orgasm).

    d. Resolution

       Resolution is a sense of well-being and general relaxation.

   3. Inhibitions may occur during one or more of these four phases of the response cycle.

   4. Sexual avoidance (phobic) is not really a psychosexual problem. Many are preoccupied with their sexual performance.

B. Prevalence

Not really known, but sexual dysfunctions are common, especially in their milder forms.

C. Etiology

   1. Women's sexual responsiveness, more than men's, tends to depend on feelings of tenderness, intimacy, affection, and security. Any factors that interfere with these underlying feelings may also impair the woman's ability to be sexually responsive.

   2. A frequent problem in the woman's impaired sexual response is the male's premature ejaculation (some say premature ejaculation in men is disappearing).

   3. Perhaps even more common is some disturbance in the total relationship with the partner.

   4. Primary male impotence usually indicates serious underlying psychopathology. Such men usually come from backgrounds of sexual repression.

   5. Men with secondary impotence are usually responding to some situational factor (e.g., excessive indulgence in alcohol, occupational or economic tensions, depression).

   6. Testosterone is the libido hormone in *both* sexes.

D. Treatment

The treatment of sexual dysfunctions has been largely influenced by the work of Masters and Johnson.

References

American Psychiatric Association. *Diagnostic and Statistical Manual of Mental Disorders.* 3d ed. Washington, D. C., 1978–1979.

Eaton, M. T., Jr.; Peterson, M. H.; and Davis, J. M. *Psychiatry.* 3d ed. Flushing, N. Y.: Medical Examination Publishing Company, 1976, chap. 15.

Farnsworth, D. L., and Braceland, F. J., eds. *Psychiatry, the Clergy and Pastoral Counseling.* Collegeville, Minn.: Saint John's University Press, 1969, chap. 20.

Freedman, A. M.; Kaplan, H. I.; and Sadock, B. J. *Modern Synopsis of Comprehensive Textbook of Psychiatry.* Vol. 2. 2d ed. Baltimore: Williams & Wilkins Company, 1976, chap. 23.

Goodwin, D.W., and Guze, S.B. *Psychiatric Diagnosis*. 2d ed. New York: Oxford University Press, 1979, chap. 12.

Hastings, D. W. *Impotence and Frigidity.* Boston: Little, Brown and Company, 1963.

Kolb, L. C. *Modern Clinical Psychiatry*. 9th ed. Philadelphia: W. B. Saunders Company, 1977, chap. 24.

Marmor, J. Sexual Deviancy: Part 1, *Journal of Continuing Education in Psychiatry,* July 1978.

————.Sexual Deviancy: Part 2, *Journal of Continuing Education in Psychiatry,* August 1978.

Masters, W. H., and Johnson, V. E. *Human Sexual Response*. Boston: Little, Brown and Company, 1966.

————.*Human Sexual Inadequacy*. Boston: Little, Brown and Company, 1970.

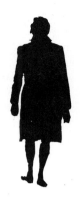

O true apothecary!
Thy drugs are quick.

Shakespeare: *Romeo and Juliet,*
Act V (c. 1596)

Substance Use Disorders

I. Introduction

A. According to the *Diagnostic and Statistical Manual of Mental Disorders,* 3d ed. (*DSM*-III), abuse of or dependence on all substances that modify mood or behavior, including alcohol, are subsumed under the category, Substance use disorders. Thus, the classification includes the abuse of alcohol, sedatives, hypnotics, opioids, cocaine, amphetamine-like drugs, hallucinogens, cannabis, phencyclidine, and even tobacco.

B. It should be kept in mind that the recreational or social use of certain drugs, such as alcohol and caffeine, is not considered abnormal.

C. The substance use disorders are subdivided into: (1) substance abuse; and (2) substance dependence.

   1. Substance abuse

   Diagnostic criteria

     a. Abuse of at least one month's duration

     b. Social complications of use (e.g., inappropriate social behavior, criminal behavior, other types of illegal activities, or difficulties in job performance)

     c. Psychological dependence (compelling desire to use the substance or to continue the use of the substance while under its influence; inability to reduce or stop use; or repeated efforts to control use by periods of temporary abstinence or restriction of use to certain times of the day)

     d. Pathological pattern of use (e.g., remaining intoxicated throughout the day, using the substance daily, or experiencing complications (e.g., alcoholic blackouts, hallucinogen delusional syndrome).

     e. Thus, there is a pattern of pathological use for at least one month and impairment in social or occupational functioning.

   2. Substance dependence

   In addition to the diagnostic criteria for substance abuse, dependence requires either

     a. Tolerance

     Tolerance means that repeated equal doses have a diminishing effect (more and more of the drug is needed to produce the effect produced by the first use), or

     b. Withdrawal symptoms

     In *withdrawal,* a substance-specific syndrome follows the cessation or reduction of the intake of the substance.

     c. Alcohol and cannabis dependence also require abuse or impairment in social or occupational functioning.

D. Classes of substances

Eight classes of substances are delineated:
1. Alcohol
2. Barbiturates or other sedatives or hypnotics
3. Opioids
4. Cocaine
5. Amphetamine or amphetamine-like compounds
6. Cannabis
7. Phencyclidine
8. Tobacco. (There is no abuse disorder because there is no clinically significant intoxication syndrome.)

E. Although abuse of alcohol technically belongs in this classification, it is being discussed in a separate chapter, since individuals who abuse alcohol often do not have other substance use disorders, whereas individuals with most other substance use disorders frequently do.

II. Prevalence

A. It is generally agreed that abuse of and dependence on drugs has increased in recent years.

B. Among adolescents, there is considerable peer pressure to experiment with various kinds of drugs.

C. The use of drugs among adolescents increased during the 1960s, but may have peaked before the close of the decade (the likely exception is the use of marijuana). Emotionally healthy, normally maturing adolescents rarely use drugs regularly.

D. Most drug-dependent people become so by their association with other people who are also drug-dependent. Their lives prior to substance use have usually been ones of unsatisfactory or marginal adjustments.

E. Medications that reduce pain, diminish anxiety, or produce euphoria may be taken by those who seek relief from physical or psychological symptoms or feelings of inadequacy.

III. Etiology

A. Many of the etiological and psychopathological factors found in substance use disorders are also associated with alcoholism (see next chapter).

B. Some drug dependence may develop after long administration of drugs for pain or other types of physical symptoms that were initially organic in origin. Such dependence has usually followed medical prescriptions of drugs by the individual's physician. In the past, this was referred to as *medical addiction*. (Medical addiction does not lead to a psychiatric diagnosis.)

C. Some people take drugs to overcome feelings of inferiority or inadequacy.
1. The individual who has reduced tolerance to tension, feelings of inadequacy, and who feels under personal or social stress may take drugs.
2. The availability of drugs and other cultural factors may play a role. Physicians are apt to abuse narcotics and barbiturates; housewives are most likely to abuse sedatives and antianxiety agents; adolescents are most apt to abuse marijuana or other street drugs. (As a matter of fact, availability of drugs is the most common predisposing factor in substance use.)
D. Some take drugs mostly for the euphoric effect (e.g., cocaine or marijuana).

IV. Psychopathology
A. Persons who develop drug dependence have subnormal tolerance of tension and above-normal feelings of dependency.
B. Features of various personality disorders are often present in substance abusers. For example, some show traits of anti-social personality, others may show evidences of borderline personality or dysthymic disorder (chronic depression).
C. Abuse of certain substances, particularly cocaine, hallucinogens, and cannabis, is often associated with identification with counter-cultural life styles (*DSM*-III).
D. Some authorities believe that there is absence of a strong father-figure in the developmental histories of people who become addicts.

V. Dependency-producing drugs
The following are some of the drugs, other than alcohol, on which people can become dependent or which they can abuse.
A. Barbiturates or similar sedatives
1. In the past, barbiturates were commonly prescribed for various types of anxiety symptoms and for sedation. The introduction of nonbarbiturate sedatives reduced their use, but they have sometimes created new addictive problems (e.g., Methaqualone, Placidyl, Doriden).
2. There are two patterns of development of abuse and dependence—
a. By individuals who originally obtained the barbiturate or other sedatives by medical prescription, but have gradually increased the dose and frequency of use on their own.
b. By individuals, usually in their teens or early twenties, who obtain the substances from illicit sources.
3. Most of these drugs produce relaxation and a sense of well-being (sedation), that is very similar to the effect of alcohol.
4. Although most persons dependent on barbiturates and other sedatives can withdraw abruptly, on rare occasions abrupt withdrawal may produce convulsions or a withdrawal delirium.

5. Non-barbiturates and sedatives are of two types—
    a. The antianxiety agents, such as meprobamate (Equanil; Miltown); diazepam (Valium); and other benzodiazapines.
    b. Sedatives, such as Placidyl, Doriden, and Noludar.
6. Course
    a. There are persons who use drugs only in certain controlled ways that protect them against progression.
    b. There is a tendency for abuse to progress to dependence.
    c. A significant number of dependent users, with or without prolonged treatment, once detoxified never again abuse these substances and appear fully recovered (*DSM*-III).

B. Opioid substances
1. Dependence on opioids generally follows a period of "polydrug use."
2. Course
    a. Once the pattern is established, it usually dominates the individual's life-style.
    b. The course is a function of the context and setting of the addiction. The vast number of Americans who used heroin in Viet Nam gave up their addiction when they returned to the United States, whereas most of those who become dependent in the United States continue the opioid-dependent life-style.

C. Cocaine
1. Cocaine has a limited use in medical practice (e.g., as an anesthetic in certain types of nasal surgery).
2. It is taken either by hypodermic injection or by sniffing ("sniffing snow").
3. It produces euphoria, loquaciousness, elation, and grandiosity.
4. Somatic hallucinations, including formication (the "cocaine bug") are sometimes experienced.
5. Course
    a. The abuse of or dependence on cocaine is not as prolonged as on the barbiturates or opioids.
    b. Dependence is psychological, not physical as on barbiturates and opiates. (Thus, technically there is no dependence as defined in *DSM*-III because there is no tolerance or withdrawal syndrome.)
    c. Psychological dependence is usually associated with a marked waning of the superego.

D. Amphetamines or similar substances
1. Medical use
    a. They were first used in otolaryngology as a nasal decongestant.

b. They were also prescribed to relieve fatigue or depression, to control appetite, or to produce wakefulness in those who had to perform tasks of long duration.

c. There are far fewer legitimate medical indications for their use now, and they have come under much closer government supervision because of their widespread abuse.

2. Prevalence and course

a. These drugs are stimulants and produce euphoria.

b. Sometimes those dependent on sedatives for sleep take them to stay awake during the daytime.

c. Many people obtain them illicitly.

d. Acute paranoid psychosis may develop in people who abuse this group of drugs. A urine test for amphetamines is necessary to make the diagnosis of amphetamine intoxication, which may be clinically indistinguishable from acute paranoid schizophrenia.

E. Hallucinogens

1. Definition

a. Among this group are lysergic acid/diethylamide (LSD); mescaline (peyote) from cactus; psilocybin, from mushroom; dimethyltryptamine (DMT); STP; morning glory seeds; nutmeg; and stramonium.

b. Phencyclidine, which is sometimes referred to as an hallucinogen, rarely causes hallucinosis.

2. Effect

a. Most produce a reaction similar to hypomania and schizophrenic withdrawal (preoccupation with own thoughts and perceptions).

b. These drugs can lead to serious psychological damage.

c. Some of the adverse affects that have been reported from LSD use are:

(1) Long-term psychotic disorders

(2) Panic from a reaction to the hallucinatory experiences ("bad trip")

(3) Serious injury and even death have resulted from the delusional experiences (e.g., feelings of omnipotence or the feeling that one can fly)

(4) Long-term intellectual and emotional disorientation

(5) Flashback phenomenon, a reexperiencing of a trip without further use of the drug

F. Cannabis

1. Cannabis, or marijuana, is a leaf that grows wild in most parts of the United States and South America.

2. Medical use

a. Cannabis was previously used as a treatment for tension headache, dysmenorhea, and glaucoma.

b. It was removed from the U. S. Pharmacopoeia in 1935.

c. As of this writing (1979), it is prescribed only experimentally, but efforts are being made to have it released for the treatment of glaucoma, of nausea and other side-effects of anti-cancer drugs, and of anorexia nervosa.

3. Prevalence

It has been used in the United States since about 1920, first by members of deprived socioeconomic groups, but later by members of the middle and affluent classes as well.

4. Chronic use produces the "amotivational syndrome."

G. Phencyclidine

1. A white powder, commonly called PCP ("peace pill").

2. Although available as a veterinary anesthetic, most of the illicit supply comes from home laboratories.

3. On the "street" it is called "angel dust."

4. It is sold in powder and tablet form, both in many colors.

5. It is often sprinkled on marijuana or parsley leaves and smoked in a "joint."

6. Its use seems to be increasing. It may well be that the use of PCP is quite common among abusers of other drugs.

7. PCP is stronger than marijuana, perhaps more comparable to LSD.

8. The diagnosis of overdosage is frequently missed because the presenting symptoms often closely resemble those of an acute schizophrenic episode.

9. Some authorities feel that phenothiazines should not be used to manage a patient during the acute stage of overdose because of the anticholinergic potentiation.

H. Tobacco use disorder

1. Included in the classification of mental disorders in *DSM*-III.

2. Chronic use of tobacco has been shown to predispose the user to a number of medical diseases. The development of such diseases is directly related to the dose of the tobacco and the route or administration. Those who inhale are, in general, at greater risk (*DSM*-III).

3. Health authorities have estimated that 15 percent of the annual mortality rate in the United States is directly due to diseases caused or aggravated by the consumption of tobacco (*DSM*-III).

4. The most common tobacco-related serious physical disorders are bronchitis, emphysema, coronary artery disease, peripheral vascular disease, and a variety of cancers.

5. In *DSM*-III, the use of tobacco is considered a mental disorder:
   a. When the use of tobacco is accompanied by distress caused by the need to use it or the user has tried to stop but is unable to
   b. There is evidence of a serious tobacco-related physical disorder in an individual who is physiologically dependent upon it (i.e., the physical illness is exacerbated by tobacco use).
I. Glue sniffing
   1. Glue sniffing
      a. Found among some children who are depressed, passive-aggressive, and have a history of delinquency.
      b. The users are usually under the age of fourteen.
      c. Physiological dependence does not develop.
   2. Other sniffing
      Other substances sniffed include gasoline vapor, pure toluene, ether, and lighter fluid.

VI. Treatment
A. Treatment of the underlying personality disorder
   1. This is often extremely difficult, because the substance abuser and substance-dependent person, like the alcoholic, has reduced tolerance for tension.
   2. Psychotherapy
      a. Psychotherapy is of help in many cases.
      b. Support and reassurance are important.
      c. Group psychotherapy has been helpful in some cases.
B. Treatment of the drug dependence
   1. Self-help group
      Groups such as AA or other groups composed of drug-dependent people are often the most helpful.
   2. Withdrawal
      a. At present, most withdrawal treatment is fairly abrupt and uses the principles of supportive treatment.
      b. Supportive treatment involves
         (1) A detoxification period during which certain drugs are judiciously prescribed. The drugs include methadone (see below), chlordiazepoxide (Librium), diazepam (Valium), Sparine, or phenobarbitol. They are continued for several days after the patient has discontinued using the abused drug.
         (2) Adequate diet and fluid intake.
         (3) Often, placement in "chemical dependency units" where patients are treated much like alcoholics. Such persons often need more "attention" than other patients.

(4) A therapeutic, supportive, and reassuring attitude. The therapist avoids being judgmental or moralistic.

   c. Methadone

Methadone (Dolophine) is the drug used to treat addicts to opiate and opiate-like agents. It is administered in two ways.

(1) Methadone substitution

In this approach, the addict takes a regular dose of methadone, given orally, after which the methadone is progressively withdrawn over a period of a few days.

(2) Methadone maintenance

In this method, the methadone is prescribed indefinitely.

3. Rehabilitation of the drug-dependent person must be regarded as a long-term management problem. Refer to the next chapter, "Alcoholism," for information about follow-up treatment and rehabilitation after the patient leaves the hospital.

VII. Prognosis

A. The prognosis is often poor.

B. Relapses are common.

C. However, given someone who is well-motivated and willing to regard his or her problem as a long-term one that must be dealt with consistently over a protracted period of time, the frequency of relapses can be reduced and the periods of abstinence can be lengthened.

D. Follow-up programs such as AA, halfway houses, and other various group settings have improved the remission rate.

VIII. Case examples

A. Medical addiction

Mrs. J., a forty-year-old housewife, had suffered from migraine headaches since puberty. They had gradually increased in frequency and severity. At thirty, she began taking codeine. For a few years, this gave some relief but for five years she had been taking demerol (a synthetic narcotic drug) in increasingly larger doses. At the time of admission to the hospital, she was using 500–600 mgm. of demerol per day (the usual dose is 50 mgm). She was always very dependent on her mother. Even after her marriage, she never lived farther away from her mother than one block. She had always had a reduced tolerance of any kind of discomfort; for example, she required medication for painful menses, sinusitis, and other pain.

Although demerol was successfully withdrawn rapidly during her hospitalization, she was never fully able to face her underlying problems of dependency and unexpressed hostility. One month after discharge, she was again beginning to take demerol for her headaches.

In the foregoing case, note that the patient began taking drugs for a psychosomatic illness (migraine), that she had a reduced tolerance of discomfort, was very dependent, and was unable to express hostile feelings.

B. Self-administration

Mr. D. S., a twenty-three-year-old single male, was referred to the court's psychiatric consultant for evaluation after he had been placed in the workhouse for driving after suspension of his license and driving under the influence of drugs. These offenses occurred while he was awaiting trial on a charge of aggravated robbery.

He had received an undesirable discharge from the Marine Corps centering around his possession and use of marijuana, "at my own request." In addition, he reported, he had been court-martialed for disrespect to a noncommissioned officer and had received minor discipline for two other offenses. Concerning his use of drugs, he said that he was first "turned on" by marijuana about three years earlier, while serving with the marines. From then until the time of the arrest that brought him to the attention of the court's consultant, he had used drugs extensively. He had used LSD and other hallucinogenic drugs, but gave these up after he began to have bad trips and flashbacks. He said that he had been hospitalized in Okinawa for four days for withdrawal of hallucinogenic drugs. He suffered minor withdrawal symptoms when he was jailed for the current offenses. Chiefly, he had been "mainlining" heroin, although he also used cocaine. Throughout this whole period, he had never tried to stop smoking marijuana, although he said that for periods of up to one or two months during the preceding four years he had been able to remain off other drugs. He also admitted that he had used "speed" intravenously. He said that his "habit" was costing him $100 to $120 a day.

Mental-status examination revealed him to be somewhat anxious and superficial, and he seemed to be trying to impress the examiner by his need to be released. He admitted feeling depressed in the past when his freedom was restricted, and also sometimes from the bad effects of drugs. Although he was lucid, appropriate, and free of psychotic mentation, he said that he was aware of paranoid ideation at times in the past when he was on drugs. He also admitted having hallucinatory experiences from LSD, mescaline and, on one occasion, from "Panama marijuana." In all of these instances, he had pleasant and vivid visual and auditory sensations. His later trips had a paranoid content and would last up to five hours. Needle scars were evident over the antecubital areas of both arms. Treatment in a hospital was recommended.

References

American Psychiatric Association. *Diagnostic and Statistical Manual of Mental Disorders.* 3d ed. Washington, D. C., 1979.

Farnsworth, D. L., and Braceland, F. J., eds. *Psychiatry, the Clergy and Pastoral Counseling.* Collegeville, Minn.: Saint John's University Press, 1969, chap. 18.

Freeman, A. M.; Kaplan, H. I.; and Sadock, B. J. *Modern Synopsis of Comprehensive Textbook of Psychiatry.* Vol. 2. Baltimore: The Williams & Wilkins Company, 1976, chap. 22.

Goodwin, D. W., and Guze, S. B. *Psychiatric Diagnosis.* 2d ed. New York: Oxford University Press, 1979, chap. 8.

Kolb, L. C. *Modern Clinical Psychiatry.* 9th ed. Philadelphia: W. B. Saunders Company, 1977, chap. 26.

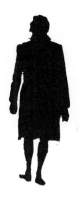

Oh, many a peer of England brews livelier liquor than the muse, and malt does more than Milton can to justify God's ways to man. Ale, man ale's the stuff to drink for fellows whom it hurts to think.

Alfred E. Housman: *A Shropshire Lad* **(1896)**

Alcoholism

I. Definition

A. *Alcoholism* is a disorder characterized by excessive use of alcohol to the point of habituation, overdependence, or addiction.

B. Many definitions of alcoholism have been formulated by various authorities, partly because of the complexity of the disorder and partly because of the divergent orientations of the investigators. Some have stressed operational aspects, while others have attempted to describe causal factors.

   1. The World Health Organization regards excessive drinking to be any form of drinking which in extent goes beyond traditional and customary use or ordinary compliance with the customs of the community. By the definition, alcoholics are those excessive drinkers whose dependence upon alcohol has attained such a degree that it causes a noticeable mental disturbance or interferes with their bodily and mental health, their interpersonal relationships, or their smooth and economic functioning.

   2. *The Manual of Alcoholism* of the American Medical Association defines alcoholism as "an illness characterized by a significant impairment that is directly associated with persistent and excessive use of alcohol. Impairment may involve physiological, psychological or social dysfunction."

   3. Alcoholics have lost the power of choice in the matter of their drinking, and their drinking interferes with their health, work, or personal relationships. Generally, one can say that persons are alcoholics if their drinking interferes in any way with their lives.

C. Technically, abuse of and dependence on alcohol belong in the chapter, "Substance Use Disorders" but, as noted there, it is being discussed separately because individuals who abuse alcohol often do not have other substance use disorders.

II. Social drinking

A. Alcohol is widely used socially. Field surveys reveal that about 71 percent of Americans drink alcohol. The rates are generally higher in urban and industrial regions. Geographically, drinking is most prevalent in the Middle Atlantic States (88 percent) and least in the East South Central Region (33 percent).

B. Today most drinking occurs in the home whereas, in the past, three-quarters of all drinking occurred in bars, taverns, pubs, and restaurants.

III. Prevalence of alcoholism

A. Not everyone who occasionally becomes drunk (or even fairly often) can be considered an alcoholic. Drinking is considered pathological only when it is prolonged and excessive.

B. No adequate prevalence rates of alcoholism are available, partly because of the lack of agreement about the definition of the disorder.
C. Of the seventy-eight million people in the United States who drink, between five to nine million are said to be alcoholics. Since most problem drinkers live with their families, it is reasonable to assume that alcoholism directly affects sixteen to twenty million Americans.
D. There are about five to six times as many male alcoholics as female alcoholics (probably because of the different role expectancies of the two sexes). This ratio has remained fairly constant in the United States for many years, even though recent estimates suggest that the proportion of female alcoholics is increasing.
E. Much of the absenteeism in industry is related to alcoholism.
F. Alcoholism is an important factor in traffic accidents, and studies have indicated that about 50 percent of fatal accidents involve alcohol abuse. In general, courts are becoming much firmer in dealing with the driver who is under the influence of alcohol.
G. Many alcoholics are unrecognized because their drinking is done secretly and their problem does not become manifest for a long time.
H. Some people who use alcohol to excess are not basically alcoholics (e.g., a person with a bipolar disorder may use alcohol excessively only when elated).
I. People who have other kinds of emotional disorders are more predisposed to alcoholism.
J. See Sociocultural factors, below.

IV. Sociocultural factors

A. Functions of alcohol
The many purposes for which various groups employ alcohol can be divided into four general categories. These purposes influence drinking patterns greatly.
1. Religious (e.g., wine in Roman Catholic and Jewish services)
2. Ceremonial (e.g., toasting the bride with champagne, drinking wine at the Bar Mitzvah ceremony)
3. Utilitarian (e.g., in cooking, medicines, as psychic balm; and at business and social functions)
4. Hedonistic (e.g., as a social lubricant and especially for the euphoria produced)[1]
B. Studies reveal low rates of alcoholism among Jews, Chinese, and Italians. Although abstinence from alcohol is uncommon in any of these groups, drunkenness is disapproved.
C. Conversely, the Irish-Americans and the French have high rates of alcoholism.

1. American Medical Association, *Manual on Alcoholism*, p. 21.

D. Studies have indicated that if persons from a Protestant background of strict abstinence drink, there is relatively high likelihood that they will become problem drinkers.

E. More men than women drink, and men drink larger amounts and more frequently. This sex difference in the rate of alcoholism is sometimes explained in terms of the different role expectancies of the two sexes. There is less social pressure on women to drink, and they are expected to drink in fewer kinds of situations. Women do not have to prove their femininity by drinking. In addition, the negative social sanctions against female drunkenness are much greater than for male drunkenness.

F. Studies of adolescent populations show that only 2 to 6 percent of the teenage users are problem drinkers.

G. Studies of industrial populations reveal that American industry numbers about two million alcoholics on its collective payroll, of whom 90 percent are in the thirty-five to fifty-five age group. Some have referred to the alcoholic in the industrial setting as the "hidden half man."

V. Etiology

A. Many theories about the etiology and psychopathology of alcoholism have been offered but the causes are not really known. Obviously, the universality of the drinking of alcohol implies that alcohol satisfies some deep-seated need in human beings. Alcohol is an effective tension-reducer.

B. The causal theories may be subsumed under two chief headings: (1) pathophysiological; and (2) psychological.

   1. Pathophysiological theories

      a. Pathophysiological theories include any approach that emphasizes hereditary, metabolic, or allergic factors and that largely ignores psychodynamic or cultural factors.

      b. Although very few authorities subscribe to pathophysiological theories, there are studies that seem to indicate some genetic predisposition toward or away from alcoholism.

      c. It has long been recognized that alcoholism is common in some families, suggesting that at least a tendency toward the disease may be inherited.

      d. It has also been proposed that inherited traits may help *ward off* alcoholism by causing unusual distress when alcohol is ingested, possibly because of excessive production of acid aldehyde during metabolism.

      e. At this point, the role of heredity is unclear.

   2. Psychological theories

   Most authorities believe that the chief causes of alcoholism are psychological.

C. Certain findings are accepted by most authorities.
  1. Drinking is common in our society, and total abstinence is rare.
  2. There are many individuals who have various types of mental disorders and many of them use alcohol.
     a. However, alcoholism is not common in most people who have these disorders.
     b. Therefore, although drinking and emotional disorder may be necessary conditions for the development of alcoholism, they cannot be regarded as sufficient conditions.
     c. Many people who have personality defects never use alcohol.
D. There are other well-accepted facts that oppose and discredit certain commonly held views.
  1. Alcohol by itself does not cause alcoholism.
  2. Alcoholism does not result from drinking a particular beverage.
  3. Alcoholism is not an allergic manifestation.
  4. Alcoholism is not due to an alcoholic personality.[2]
E. The person who uses alcohol to excess is making an attempt at self-treatment. From a psychological point of view, alcoholics are often said to
  1. Be emotionally immature
  2. Be emotionally dependent
  3. Be passive
  4. Have a reduced tolerance of anxiety (anything that reduces anxiety may become a habit)
  5. Have been brought up by overprotective and overindulgent parents who encouraged infantile oral demands
F. Drinking often makes it easier to express feelings of rejection, dependency, or sexuality. This can lead to remorse and guilt that, in turn, make it easy for the individual to drink to relieve these symptoms, too.
G. From the psychoanalytic viewpoint
  1. Alcoholism has been regarded as a reaction to latent homosexuality. However, many authorities now believe that the male alcoholic's avoidance of relationships with the opposite sex and preference for the company of his own sex most likely represent a striving for a simple, noninvolving type of relationship.
  2. The alcoholic has a narcissistic premorbid personality and, under the influence of alcohol, allows himself or herself to return to a kind of omnipotent state, unhampered by the realities of the external world, believing that anything is possible, and that he or she is great and can do anything.
  3. Conflicts or trauma during the oral phase of development are considered to be of etiological significance.

2. *Manual On Alcoholism*, pp. 9–11.

H. Drinking among alcoholics seems to be based largely on unconscious rather than conscious factors, and the goal of drinking seems to be to establish psychodynamic equilibrium in dealing with stresses.

I. The course of alcoholism seems different for the two sexes. Serious dependence on alcohol occurs about a decade later in women. Women alcoholics are much more likely to have a history of affective disorder.

J. Cultural-anthropological theories
This approach stresses the influence of diverse cultural and social pressures. Evidence includes—
   1. The capacity for alcoholic consumption is equated with masculinity or toughness; young men start drinking as a way of conforming to the ways of the peer group.
   2. Rates of alcoholism are higher in urban populations.

K. Alcoholism is, however, found in virtually all socioeconomic groups.

L. In general, the underlying etiology of alcoholism is similar to that of many other types of mental disorders.

M. In summary, alcoholism should probably be regarded as resulting from a complex interaction of psychological, sociocultural, biological, and possibly genetic factors. An eclectic and empirical approach to this problem is indicated.

N. In the chronic stage, it is important to keep in mind that alcoholism should be regarded as a symptom that itself has become a disease.

VI. Psychopathology

A. Alcoholics lack some ego-strength and, like persons with character defects, are unable to control their impulses.

B. They have difficulty tolerating tension. This is sometimes thought to be related to their inconsistent training in dealing with reality.

C. They are dependent. This seems related to difficulties in their very early development (the oral period, according to psychoanalytic theory).

D. They are usually passive.

E. They often seem socially uneasy.

VII. Symptomatology

A. Some alcoholics have symptoms of other emotional disorders (e.g., anxiety or depression).

B. Some alcoholics have symptoms of character defects (e.g., antisocial or passive-aggressive personality).

C. Others seem to have no obvious symptom apart from the excessive drinking.

D. Toxic effects may accompany alcoholism (see IX, this chapter).

E. The defenses that seem most common among alcoholics are
   1. Rationalization
   2. Denial
   3. Projection
F. Patterns
   1. Some alcoholics are spree, or periodic drinkers; that is, they drink excessively for a period of time. Included in this group are those who plan drinking episodes carefully.
   2. Others are continual drinkers. Such alcoholics sip every day and, though never obviously intoxicated, are nearly always under the influence of alcohol.
   3. Some alcoholics restrict their drinking to weekends.
G. Some authorities divide alcoholism into
   1. Essential alcoholism
      Included here are those people who have drifted across the line from social drinking without any other obvious emotional problems. Also known as *addictive drinking, compulsive drinking,* and *alcoholism simplex.*
   2. Symptomatic alcoholism
      The drinking is a symptom of a serious emotional disorder, such as anxiety disorder, affective disorder, or schizophrenic disorder.
   3. Reactive drinking
      Drinking in response to some particular emotional stress such as the death of a loved one; the alcohol helps the individual "work through" his or her feelings of grief.
H. Seldon Bacon has given three criteria for determining the presence of alcoholism in individuals:
   1. They not only ingest more alcohol, but in different ways from their appropriate associates.
   2. So-called problems, especially of an intrapersonal and emotional nature, that are clearly related to the deviant use of alcohol emerge chronically.
   3. There is a growing loss of rational, socially mature self-control over the ingestion of alcohol.

VIII. Course
The progression into alcoholism often proceeds as follows.
A. The drinking is at first social and masquerades as a companionable or relaxing activity.
B. Then the drinkers turn to alcohol for escape from stress and anxiety and feelings of inadequacy.
C. Later, their self-control diminishes and their need for alcohol increases.

D. As control lessens, their work begins to suffer, and so also does their health, family and social relationships, and all other aspects of their lives.

IX. Toxic alcoholic syndromes

A. Alcohol intoxication

In the *Diagnostic and Statistical Manual of Mental Disorders, 3d ed.* (*DSM*-III) *alcohol intoxication* is defined as simple intoxication. The essential features are slurred speech, incoordination, unsteady gait and impairment of memory. Psychological signs include mood liability, irritability, loquacity, loss of inhibition of sexual and aggressive impulses. The person may engage in certain other kinds of maladaptive behavior, such as fighting, or suffer from impaired judgment, impaired social or occupational functioning, and failure to meet responsibilities. Personality traits may be exaggerated; thus, the drinker may become depressed, euphoric, manic, paranoid, or expansive (*DSM*-III).

B. Alcohol idiosyncratic intoxication

Alcohol idiosyncratic intoxication is pathological intoxication. It is characterized by overreaction to minimal amounts of alcohol, less than sufficient to cause intoxication in most people. The onset of marked behavioral changes, while drinking or shortly thereafter, is sudden and dramatic, and it frequently involves aggressive behavior that is atypical of the person when not drinking (*DSM*-III).

C. Alcohol withdrawal

Alcohol withdrawal is the development of withdrawal symptoms shortly after not drinking for several days or longer. Characterized by tremors of the hand, tongue, and eyelids, and by associated symptoms such as nausea and vomiting, malaise or weakness, autonomic hyperactivity (e.g., tachycardia, sweating, elevated blood pressure), anxiety, depressed mood or irritability, insomnia, grand mal seizures, or orthostatic hypotension (*DSM*-III).

D. Alcohol withdrawal delirium

Alcohol withdrawal delirium, or *delirium tremens,* is an acute psychotic episode occurring within one week after the cessation or reduction of heavy alcohol intake, characterized by delirium, coarse tremors, and perceptual disturbances, including illusions and frightening visual hallucinations that usually become more intense in the dark. The cause of the condition is not definitely known, but is thought to be a metabolic disturbance (*DSM*-III).

1. The hallucinations are vivid, most commonly visual, and usually colorful. Tactile and olfactory hallucinations are also fairly common. Auditory hallucinations are rare. Delusions are in keeping with the hallucinations. The patient is usually overactive and may be irritable, but is sometimes silly or euphoric.

2. The tremors may be generalized or limited to groups of muscles (*DSM*-III).
E. Alcohol hallucinosis
   Alcohol hallucinosis is hallucinosis that persists after a person has recovered from the symptoms of alcohol withdrawal and is no longer drinking. The hallucinations usually begin one to two weeks after the cessation of drinking. There is some controversy about whether this is a discrete syndrome or a manifestation of another psychiatric disorder in an individual who was incidentally a heavy drinker (*DSM*-III).
F. Alcohol amnestic syndrome
   Alcohol amnestic syndrome is known as *Korsakoff's syndrome.* The essential feature is an irreversible amnesia associated with disorientation, confabulation, and peripheral neuropathy. It is associated with chronic alcoholism and is believed due to a nutritional deficiency, particularly of thiamine and niacin.
   1. There is delirium of a mild degree, defects in memory and retention, and disorientation.
   2. Confabulation, the invention of an imaginary experience to fill in memory gaps, is typical.
   3. Peripheral neuropathy is most marked in the lower extremities (*DSM*-III).
G. Wernicke's syndrome
   Wernicke's syndrome is a rare disorder of central-nervous-system metabolism, associated with a thiamine deficiency and seen chiefly in chronic alcoholics. It is characterized by irregular eye movements, incoordination, impaired thinking and, often, sensory-motor deficit. Korsakoff's psychosis, with accompanying confabulation, commonly accompanies Wernicke's syndrome.
H. Dementia associated with alcoholism
   Dementia associated with alcoholism is found in patients with a history of alcoholism who demonstrate the features of dementia (deterioration) even when they are not intoxicated or undergoing withdrawal. Dementia associated with alcoholism may be a consequence of alcohol or an indirect result of malnutrition. In *DSM*-II, this disorder was called *alcoholic deterioration.*

X. **Treatment**
A. Treatment of the underlying personality disorder
   1. Pharmacological treatment
      a. Aversion therapy
         Aversion therapy, in which a conditioned response is established, is rarely used now.

b. Disulfram therapy

This is the antabuse treatment. Following its introduction in 1948, this therapy gained wide acceptance, but it, too, seems to have had only limited use in the treatment of alcoholism. The drug, tetraethylthiurium disulfide, when combined with alcohol, produces distressing vasomotor symptoms. Unlike the aversion treatment, no conditioned response is established; the unpleasant effects are produced by mixing antabuse and alcohol. The patients must take the antabuse each day: if they stop for several days, they can drink alcohol without the distressing symptoms. Patients who receive this treatment must be in good physical health. Special examinations of the heart, liver, and kidneys are often performed before the drug is administered.

　　　c. Tranquilizing drugs

Various types of psychotropic drugs are sometimes helpful in the management of alcoholism, either for facilitating psychotherapy or for mitigating anxiety or the symptoms of overindulgence. Neuroleptics are also used in the management of acute psychotic conditions related to alcoholic excesses. Among the tranquilizing medications that have been used in alcoholism are chlordiazepoxide (Librium), diazepam (Valium), chlorpromazine (Thorazine), and promazine (Sparine).

2. Psychotropic drugs

Various types of psychotropic drugs may be indicated when there is psychiatric disorder. The drug should be appropriate to the underlying disorder. For example, phenothiazines such as Thorazine, Stelazine, or Mellaril are used when there are overt or nearly overt psychotic processes. Antianxiety agents, including meprobamate (Equanil and Miltown) and the benzodiazepines derivatives such as Valium and Librium, are rarely prescribed for these patients, and then only with great caution, because of the possibility of creating dependence.

3. Hospitalization

　　　a. Hospitalization is often indicated. It provides a neutral and protected environment in which psychotherapy may be attempted. Hospitalization is often necessary to help alcoholics to begin a period of abstinence, as well as help them through withdrawal (detoxification).

　　　b. Patients are often hospitalized in a "chemical dependency unit." In many parts of the country, special programs have been set up for the treatment of alcoholism and other drug dependencies. These are exclusively for treatment of "the chemically dependent" (patients with substance use disorders), are usually not under the direction of a psychiatrist, and usually do not have a psychiatric consultant. The personnel who run these programs are often people who have had substance use disorders themselves.

4. Psychotherapy
   a. Any psychotherapeutic approach must operate from the premise that alcoholism is a personality problem and not a moral one.
   b. The ideal treatment goal should be the elimination of the desire to drink, rather than restraint.
   c. It is also important to keep in mind that the alcoholic is usually a dependent person who often has hostile, anxious, and guilty feelings.
   d. Psychotherapy has had only limited success, one reason being that the uncovering of conflicts produces anxiety, whereas the alcoholic has a reduced tolerance of tension.
   e. Certain authorities emphasize the importance of "surrender" versus submission in any psychotherapeutic approach; that is, the alcoholics must *accept* the fact that they are alcoholics, and not just admit it.

5. Group therapy
   Group therapy is often useful in the treatment of alcoholics. Sometimes, but not always, such therapy is moderated by a professional person, such as a psychiatrist, clinical psychologist, or social worker.

6. Community resources
   a. Continued care following discharge from the hospital or a chemical dependency unit is crucial. It is true that a "supportive network" is needed by all alcoholics, but it is especially necessary for those who lack close personal relationships. It is also important to keep in mind that the family, or other people affected by the alcoholic's disorder, may also need assistance.
   b. There are many agencies and organizations concerned with this problem.
      (1) The National Institute on Alcohol Abuse and Alcoholism, P. O. Box 2345, Rockville, Maryland (part of the Alcohol, Drug Abuse and Mental Health Administration of the U. S. Department of Health and Human Services). This organization provides funds to encourage the development of programs and makes research grants to investigators and institutions studying the disorder. It also conducts educational programs at the national level and is a source of valuable information for those working in the field.

(2) Most states have a department for alcoholism or substance use disorder.

(3) In many communities there is an alcoholism information center that acts as the coordinator of available resources for the understanding and treatment of alcohol problems.

c. Alcoholics Anonymous (AA) is an informal worldwide fellowship of groups of alcoholics who help each other to stay sober and to remain abstinent. The basic philosophy is based on twelve steps and twelve traditions. The basic source of AA's strength is the relationship with God as the individual understands Him. For those who fit well into formal group activity, this approach has proven effective in maintaining sobriety. Of all the available resources, it has easily been the most helpful. However, there are some who cannot accept this approach, particularly those who have difficulty accepting a personal God.

Various attempts have been made to explain why the program has been so useful. Some think the evangelistic theme and religious overtones are important; others view the program as a resocialization process. Most local AA groups have telephone listings and place referral information in the personal columns in the newspapers.

d. Alanon and Alateen cater to the "significant others" in the alcoholic's life, who often need help to understand the problem and also to help the recovering alcoholic to maintain his or her health and sobriety. These people are sometimes referred to as "near" or "co-alcoholics."

e. Since the decriminalization of drunkenness and the enactment of the Uniform Alcoholism and Intoxication and Treatment Act of 1970, detoxification centers for the treatment of alcoholics have been established in many communities. One significant advantage of such a place is that it is usually tied into the therapeutic network for alcoholics.

f. Many communities have established various types of halfway houses where alcoholics who have no place to live may go to avoid a life-style that is conducive to drinking. Such halfway houses usually have various support groups, including local AA groups.

g. Many churches and religious groups sponsor other active programs. Among them are Calix, a group for Catholic alcoholics, and social agencies such as the Salvation Army. The local mental health association is also a possible source of information.

B. Treatment of the toxic syndromes
  1. Treatment of acute psychotic reactions
     a. Hospitalization and withdrawal of alcohol. In the past, withdrawal was sometimes gradual in order to mitigate the delirious symptoms, but most withdrawal is now abrupt.
     b. Maintaining adequate nutrition, fluid, and electrolyte intake. Use of intravenous fluids is usually not indicated, since chronic alcoholics usually are already overhydrated.
     c. Adequate vitamin intake, especially thiamine and niacin. These can be administered parenterally or orally, as indicated.
     d. Psychotropic drugs. Medications are often useful in the management of withdrawal of alcohol. Among these are chlordiazepoxide (Librium) and promazine (Sparine). If a withdrawal seizure is anticipated, an anticonvulsant such as Dilantin may be added.
     e. Corticotropin. Used intramuscularly or intravenously, this drug has been helpful in many cases of acute hallucinosis or delirium tremens.
  2. Treatment of the chronic mental disorders secondary to alcoholism
     a. Hospitalization is often necessary, sometimes permanently.
     b. Intake of fluids, vitamins, and so forth is maintained.
     c. Various psychotropic drugs may help to relieve certain symptoms. Antidepressants are used to relieve depression; antipsychotic agents are used if there is psychotic behavior.
     d. Since the brain damage is irreversible, treatment is only palliative.

XI. Prevention
  A. Alcoholism is one of the four major public-health concerns in the United States (the others are mental disorders, cardiovascular disease, and cancer).
  B. There is a need to identify and discover cases of alcoholism *early* if we are to make any progress in controlling this disorder. Case findings should be active rather than passive. Many of the community programs, including those in industry, have this orientation.
  C. Very little is known about the prevention of alcoholism.
  D. Research in social, psychological, and biological areas is a continuing need.
  E. The United States government has created the National Institute on Alcohol Abuse and Alcoholism, a major, federally funded program to prevent and control alcoholism. It works closely with the various states.

XII. Case examples

A. Alcoholism with hallucinations

J. P. C., a thirty-eight-year-old single man, was referred to the court's psychiatric consultant for evaluation after he had pleaded guilty to a charge of drunkenness, growing out of an incident in which he was arrested for behaving in a strange manner near a neighbor's apartment building. When questioned by the police who were called, he said he was looking for his sister who was in a tree. He said that he had dropped her child in a culvert and that he had retrieved the baby. He explained that his sister, while changing the baby's diaper, was snatched up into the tree. The man appeared to be intoxicated and admitted to the officers that he had been drinking.

When interviewed by the psychiatric consultant, he admitted that he had been drinking excessively for years. For about a week before his arrest, he was aware that he was "acting screwy," that is, imagining things, but whenever he ceased drinking temporarily, he hallucinated. For example, he recalled that he believed that two men had crawled through the transom of his room at a cheap downtown hotel. This was so real that he phoned the police to complain.

Following his arrest, he experienced other vivid hallucinations. For example, he thought there were cockroaches in his cell and that the jailer was throwing ants into his cell to eat the cockroaches. In addition, he was certain that he had seen his drinking companion in jail with him and he insisted, when he was bailed out by his brother, that the companion was still there (which was not true).

His background history revealed that he had been arrested about twenty times, mostly for drinking, including one arrest for drunken driving and another for petit theft committed while he was drinking. He had been hospitalized on three occasions for his drinking problem. He believed that his drinking had been a serious problem for at least thirteen or fourteen years and said, "It continually gets worse." He had been in Alcoholics Anonymous programs at various times, but regarded it as a married man's organization and considered it populated by many people who were not really alcoholics.

In addition, he complained of nervousness, uneasiness, and anxiety which, he said, antedated his first drinking. His Minnesota Multiphasic Personality Inventory profile revealed a high level of anxiety and indicated that he was worried, apprehensive, and tense.

He admitted to a very poor employment record over the years because of his drinking problem, and had been unemployed for six months prior to his arrest. For approximately a year before that, he had worked as an unskilled laborer.

This case is one of severe, chronic alcoholism in which the person also has symptoms of an anxiety disorder. In addition, he experienced a bout of acute alcoholic hallucinosis which brought him to the attention of the police. The prognosis is poor.

B. Alcoholism with depression

C. T., a fifty-two-year-old woman, was admitted to the hospital, at the request of her personal physician, for depression and a drinking problem. Her husband, who brought her to the hospital, reported that when he returned home from a business trip, he found his wife drunk and she said she was unable to control her compulsive drinking. Her physician was summoned and arrangements were made for her admission to the hospital.

Her background history revealed that she had always been a passive person and had difficulty with recurrent depressive feelings. She had made two suicide attempts, once with barbiturates, and, on another occasion, with carbon monoxide in her automobile. She had been hospitalized for psychiatric treatment on at least four other occasions.

Prominent among her symptoms while she was in the hospital were social uneasiness and the ease with which she could feel rejected. Feelings of dependency, inferiority, and inadequacy were also evident. She said that, for a number of years while she was struggling with her depressed feelings and her compulsion to drink, she blamed her difficulty on her husband. About three or four years earlier, she had finally come to realize that the problem was within her and not the fault of her husband. She had gone to AA meetings a number of times but, because of her passivity, she did not follow through very faithfully.

In this case, alcoholism complicates a recurrent depressive reaction. She was placed on antidepressants and psychotherapy and was referred to a local AA group for supportive help. A follow-up evaluation, six months following her discharge from the hospital, revealed that she had done reasonably well and had had only three minor slips, when she drank a few beers over a one- or two-day period.

References

American Medical Association. *Manual on Alcoholism.* 3d ed. Chicago, 1977.

American Psychiatric Association. *Diagnostic and Statistical Manual of Mental Disorders.* 3d ed. Washington, D. C., 1979.

Bacon, Seldon D. "The Interrelatedness of Alcoholism and Marital Conflicts." *American Journal Of Psychiatry* XXIX (1959): 153.

Farnsworth, D. L., and Braceland, F. J., eds. *Psychiatry, the Clergy and Pastoral Counseling.* Collegeville, Minn.: Saint John's University Press, 1969, chap. 17.

Goodwin, D. W., and Guze, S. B. *Psychiatric Diagnosis.* 2d ed. New York: Oxford University Press, 1979, chap 7.

Jellinek, E. M. *The Disease Concept of Alcoholism.* Highland Park, N. J.: Hillhouse Press, 1960.

Keller, M. "The Definition of Alcoholism and the Estimation of Its Prevalence." In *Society, Culture and Drinking Patterns,* edited by D. D. J. Pittman and C. R. Snyder. New York: John Wiley & Sons, 1962, chap. 17.

Mendelson, J. H., ed. *Alcoholism.* Boston: Little, Brown and Company, 1966.

World Health Organization, Expert Committee on Alcohol. *First Report.* W. H. O. Technical Report Series, no. 84, Geneva, 1955.

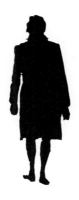

Adjustment Disorders

Mankind is made up of inconsistencies, and no man acts invariably up to his predominant character.
The wisest man sometimes acts weakly and the weakest sometimes wisely.

Philip Dormer Stanhope, 4th Earl of Chesterfield: *Letters to his Son* **(1748)**

I. Definition

According to the *Diagnostic and Statistical Manual of Mental Disorders, 3d edition (DSM*-III), the essential feature of adjustment disorder is a maladaptive reaction to an identifiable life event or circumstance that is not merely an exacerbation of one of the mental disorders previously described and that is expected to remit if and when the stressor ceases. The maladaptive nature of the reaction is indicated by the presence of either (a) impairment of social or occupational functioning; or (b) symptoms of other behavior in excess of the normal and expectable reaction to the stressor.

II. The stressors

A. Stressors may be single (e.g., an uncomplicated divorce) or multiple (e.g., the death of a loved one at a time of marked business difficulties and physical illness) [*DSM*-III].

B. The severity of the disorder is not directly related to the severity of the stressors.

III. Subtypes

This disorder may manifest itself in a number of ways, hence there are several different subtypes, including

A. Adjustment disorder with depressed mood

B. Adjustment disorder with anxious mood

C. Adjustment disorder with mixed emotional features

D. Adjustment disorder with disturbance of conduct

E. Adjustment disorder with mixed disturbance of emotions and conduct

F. Adjustment disorder with withdrawal

G. Adjustment disorder with work (or academic) inhibition

IV. Prevalence

A. This disorder is apparently quite common.

B. It may occur at any age.

V. Onset and course

A. The onset may be either immediate or delayed, and either sudden or gradual.

B. The disorder usually remits when the stressor ceases.

References

American Psychiatric Association. *Diagnostic and Statistical Manual of Mental Disorders.* 3d ed. Washington, D. C., 1979.

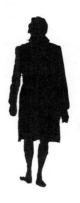

Affective Disorders

Hence, loathed melancholy,
Of Cerberus and blackist midnight
  born,
In Stygian cave forelorn,
'Mongst horrid shapes, and shrieks
  and sights unholy!

John Milton: *L'Allegro* **(1632)**

I. Introduction

A. The term *affective disorder* is a general one and refers to a mental disorder in which fundamental disturbance is in the mood.

B. The mood changes—to depression or elation—differ from other mood swings chiefly in degree and duration. The change may occur without apparent cause, seem disproportionate, or persist too long.

C. Any concomitant disturbances in thought or behavior are appropriate to the mood.

D. The disorders grouped here include those which, in previous classifications of the American Psychiatric Association, were grouped in various categories, including (1) affective disorders; (2) personality disorders; and (3) neurotic disorders.

E. In recent years, much research has been concerned with these disorders. Improvements have been made in various drug treatments, including the tricyclic antidepressants, monoamine oxidase inhibitors, Lithium, and some of the neuroleptics. (For details, see Pharmacotherapy, in the chapter, "Treatment in Psychiatry.")

II. Clinical types

A. Cases of affective disorder really fall along a continuum varying from mild, short-lived, subclinical depressions and elations on one end, to severe delusional depressions and delirious manias on the other.

B. In the 3d edition of the *Diagnostic and Statistical Manual of Mental Disorders* (*DSM*-III), the affective disorders are classified as follows:

  1. Major affective disorders
    a. Bipolar disorder
      (1) Mixed
      (2) Manic
      (3) Depressed
    b. Major depression
      (1) Single episode
      (2) Recurrent
  2. Other specific affective disorders
    a. Cyclothymic disorder
    b. Dysthymic disorder (depressive neurosis)
  3. Atypical affective disorders
    a. Atypical bipolar disorder
    b. Atypical depression.

C. In *DSM*-III, the former terms—*manic depressive illness, involutional melancholia, psychotic depressive reaction,* and *depressive neurosis*—have been dropped. Manic depressive illness is now classed as a bipolar affective disorder; involutional melancholia and psychotic depressive reaction are considered major depressive disorders; and some of the neurotic depressions are considered major depressive disorders while others would probably now be included under the term dysthymic disorder.

III. Degrees of depression

A. Normal depression

Feelings of sadness, disappointment, despair, frustration, or unhappiness are universally experienced. Such depression is considered a normal feeling state.

B. Grief (uncomplicated bereavement)

Bereavement is a normal, appropriate, affective sadness in response to a recognizable external loss. It is realistic and appropriate to what has been lost; it is self-limiting and gradually subsides. It seldom leads to serious disorder in one's personal life.

C. Mild depression (dysthymic disorder)

The etiologic factor in mild depression is less obvious than in normal grief, or the depression is more severe, or it persists unduly. The situation that occasions the reaction is often more of a precipitating event than a causal factor. The individual usually realizes that the response is excessive, but does not recognize the underlying cause.

D. Major depression (psychotic depression)

This type of depression is so profound that the patient may lose contact with reality, develop delusions, and is frequently a serious suicidal risk.

IV. Symptoms

A. There are certain symptoms that are usually found in any type of depression. These vary according to the type and severity of the depression.

1. Disturbed sleep

May be manifested as difficulty in falling asleep, difficulty in staying asleep, or early morning awakening.

2. Disturbed appetite

May be diminished interest in food, absence of appetite, or refusal to eat for delusional reasons.

3. Somatic symptoms

May be manifested as mild responses of the autonomic nervous system, which innervates the cardiovascular, digestive, reproductive, and respiratory systems; hypochondriacal preoccupation; or definite physical symptoms or somatic delusions. Often, it is the somatic symptom which first concerns the patient and leads her or him to seek medical examination.

4. In addition, the individual often feels better in the evening than in the morning (there is no good explanation for this).

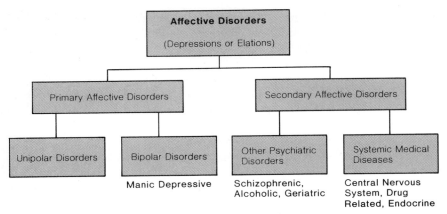

Adapted from Gerald L. Klerman, In "Affective Disorders." In *The Harvard Guide to Modern Psychiatry,* A. M. Nicholi, Ed., copyright © 1978 by Harvard University Press. Used by permission of the publishers.

V. Clinical types of depression

Robbins et al. have divided affective disorders into primary and secondary.

  A. *Primary affective disorders* are those that occur in persons who have never had an episode before or whose only previous psychiatric illnesses were episodes of depression or mania.

  B. *Secondary affective disorders* occur in persons who have had other psychiatric illnesses (e.g., schizophrenia or alcoholism) or who have suffered an affective disorder related to a medical condition.

VI. Descriptive types of depression

  A. Aside from the official diagnostic classification of the various depressive disorders, certain clinical types of depression are often described.

  B. It should be kept in mind that depression is really a syndrome and that modern researchers suggest multiple etiologies.

  C. Symptom complex (subtypes)

    1. Bipolar-unipolar dichotomy

      a. The *bipolar* group consists of patients who have had both depressive and manic episodes.

      b. The *unipolar* group is those who have only had depressive episodes.

      c. Genetic studies indicate that persons with a bipolar affective disorder have families with a greater frequency of a similar illness.

      d. Patients with bipolar disorders are more likely to have hypomanic responses to tricyclic antidepressants.

    2. The psychotic-neurotic dichotomy

      a. This distinction has lost its importance in recent years.

b. The frequency of depressions of psychotic proportions has greatly decreased in recent years. Perhaps this is in part accounted for by the fact that people with signs of depression receive early treatment; hence, the fully developed psychotic syndromes described in the past do not occur.
3. Endogenous-reactive dichotomy
   This subdivision of depression is based on whether or not the depression seemed to develop "from within" (*endogenous*) or was related to life events (*reactive*). (Melancholia is synonymous with endogenous.)
4. Agitated-retarded dichotomy
   This subdivision is based on whether or not the symptoms include
   a. Uneasiness, mental perturbation, and motor restlessness (agitation),
   b. Slowing down of mental and physical activity (retardation).
5. Primary-secondary dichotomy
   (See IV)
6. Early vs. late onset
   This includes, "pure" vs. "spectrum" depression, involutional depression, chronic characterological depression, and hysteroid dysphoria.
7. Life events and stress as precipitating factors
   a. Not all persons who experience loss and separation subsequently develop depression.
   b. Loss and separation are demonstrable in only about a quarter of people with depressions.
   c. Loss and separation may precipitate a wide variety of psychiatric conditions.
   d. Predisposing factors, as well as precipitating factors, must be taken into account. Genetic factors (e.g., in the bipolar affective disorder) or early life experiences may render the individual sensitive to losses or separations.

VII. Suicide
   A. Introductory comments
      1. Since the possibility of suicide is frequently raised by depressive disorders of all types, it is considered here.
      2. However, it should be kept in mind that suicide is not exclusively limited to people with such diagnoses. Nearly everyone has had death wishes and suicidal thoughts.
      3. The number of suicidal attempts is much smaller than the number of people who have contemplated suicide, and the percentage of successful suicides is even smaller. It is variously estimated that attempts are five to fifty times more common than successes (the most common estimate seems to be ten attempts for every successful suicide).

B. Prevalence
   1. Suicide is the tenth major cause of death in the United States. Among white males, aged fifteen to nineteen, it is the second major cause of death.
   2. According to Schneidman, suicide accounts for 2,200 to 5,000 deaths annually in the United States, although the actual figure may be double.
   3. Some studies indicate that it is rare for people to make more than one suicide attempt.
   4. Although more attempts are made by women in the United States, more men are successful.
   5. Sociocultural influences
      a. Suicide is less common in Catholic countries, such as Ireland, and more common in Japan, Germany, Denmark, and Switzerland.
      b. Cultural attitudes toward suicide, death, and afterlife seem to play a role.
   6. Suicide prevention centers have apparently not affected the suicide rate.
C. Psychodynamic factors
   1. Most authorities believe that suicide rarely results from a single cause. Several factors may be operant in a cumulative way.
   2. Any serious loss may be a possible etiological factor (e.g., loss of a loved one, a job, money, health, beauty, independence).
   3. The anniversary of an important event (e.g., the death of a loved one) may initiate a suicide attempt.
   4. Karl Menninger regarded suicide as self-murder. In *Man against Himself,* he also described other self-destructive behavior that stops short of suicide (invalidism, alcoholism, self-mutilation, and accident proneness).
   5. Beck was not able to substantiate the earlier dynamic formulation of internalized aggression.
   6. Schneidman and Farberow have classified people who commit suicide into four general groups—
      a. Those who view suicide as a means to a better life or as a means of saving reputation
      b. Those who are psychotic and commit suicide in response to delusions or hallucinations
      c. Those who commit suicide as revenge against a loved person
      d. Elderly and infirm people who use suicide as a release from pain
   7. What prods a person from contemplation to action is not really known.

8. Some authorities feel that suicide attempts are motivated by
   a. A wish for revenge
   b. Feelings of hopelessness
   c. Fantasies of reunion (anniversary suicide)
   d. Thus, suicide contains a wish to kill as well as a wish to die. Hostility toward rejecting persons, presumed or actual, may motivate individuals to attempt to kill themselves and thus make the rejecting person feel guilty.
D. Danger signs
   1. History of previous suicide attempts or threats
   2. Suicide note
   3. Psychotic reactions with suspiciousness, paranoid delusions, or panic
   4. Chronic illness (especially the attitude toward the illness)
   5. Alcoholism or drug dependency
   6. Advancing age, especially in men
   7. Recent surgery or childbirth
   8. Hypochondriasis
   9. Unaccepted homosexuality
E. Evaluation of suicidal risks.
   Most suicidal patients will admit their intentions to a physician. When estimating the possibility that a person will attempt suicide, the following questions are helpful.
   1. Have you thought of suicide?
   2. Have you thought of what way you would take your life?
   3. Have you already made preparations?
   4. Do you trust yourself?

VIII. Symptomatology of affective disorders
A. Depression
   1. The chief clinical complaints of patients with depression are psychological.
      a. Depressed mood
         The patient has a feeling of sadness, gloominess, dejection, hopelessness, despondency.
         (1) The vast majority of depressed patients complain of this.
         (2) Behavior is consistent with the verbally expresssed depression.
         (3) A small number of patients do not spontaneously complain of depression, but the disorder is manifested as two other symptom complexes. Such covert depression may appear as
            (a) Chiefly hypochondriacal symptoms
            (b) Neurasthenic symptoms of exhaustion, fatigue, or weakness

(4) A few cases are "smiling depression."

(5) The complaint may be pleasurelessness (anhedonia). Previous interests no longer gratify the patient.

b. Anorexia

Most depressed patients suffer loss of appetite and often lose weight. A small number, usually adolescents, have increased appetite (bulimia).

c. Insomnia

Most patients experience some type of sleep disturbance. This may involve difficulty falling asleep, difficulty staying asleep, or early morning awakening. A few, usually adolescents, sleep excessively (hypersomnia).

d. Psychomotor retardation or psychomotor agitation

Depressive patients may appear retarded or agitated.

(1) Retarded depressions are manifested by decreased activity—

(a) Slowed speech and verbal frugality

(b) Inactivity; in stuporous depression, the patient may be mute, immobile, and severely regressed

(2) Agitated depressions are manifested by increased psychomotor activity—

(a) Restlessness, jitteriness, pacing, wringing of the hands

(b) Difficulty in concentration—the patient reports that thinking is slowed down or that his or her mind is a blank, and he often complains of loss of memory

e. Anxiety

(1) Many depressed patients complain of tension—i.e., apprehension, tension, or uneasiness.

(2) This symptom is to be distinguished from agitation, since the latter responds to neuroleptic agents, whereas anxiety responds to benzodiazepines.

f. Lowered self-esteem

Lowered self-esteem is accompanied by feelings of inadequacy, incompetence, and poor self-concept.

g. Diminished sexual interests

This symptom is common during depressions, but not offered as a presenting symptom. Depressed men are sometimes impotent.

h. Diurnal variations

Many feel better in the evening than in the morning.

i. Suicidal thoughts

Many patients have suicidal thoughts, but only a few have suicidal urges.

2. Somatic symptoms
    a. These may be manifested as a mild physiological response of any body system, hypochondriacal preoccupation, definite physical symptoms, or somatic delusions.
    b. Often it is the somatic symptom that first concerns the patients and leads them to seek medical examination.
    c. Thus, depressed persons may complain of any one of a variety of physical complaints, such as headache, cramps, nausea, constipation, or indigestion.
3. Depression as a syndrome
    a. A depressed patient usually has a constellation of the above-mentioned symptoms, but does not manifest all of them.
    b. Thus, we may speak of three depressive syndromes—
        (1) Ideational depressions (depressed mental content and few if any physical or motor symptoms)
        (2) Retarded depressions
        (3) Agitated depressions
B. Mania
1. In general, mania is characterized by flight of ideas, elated or grandiose mood, and psychomotor excitement (generalized physical and emotional overactivity). The individual with manic excitement seems to be running away from recurrent depression (cyclothymic personality or cyclothymia).
2. Elations are manifested on a continuum from hypomania to delirious mania. They are far less frequent than depressions.
    a. Cyclothymic disorder (cyclothymic personality or cyclothymia): a disorder characterized by recurring and alternating periods of depression and elation not readily attributable to external circumstances.
    b. Hypomania (mild mania)
        (1) *Hypomania* is characterized by increased happiness or optimism.
        (2) In hypomania, the thought process, rather than its content, is disturbed. Each individual act seems normal, but when it is considered together with other acts, the patient's deviation becomes evident.
        (3) Characteristically,
            (a) The patients are active, ebullient, socially aggressive, talkative, boisterous, and flippant.
            (b) They behave with heightened emotional tone; they are effusive and euphoric.
            (c) They are impatient and become irritable when frustrated.
            (d) They are superficial and insensitive in relationships with others.
            (e) They are intolerant of criticism.

(f) They are distractible (respond quickly to stimuli, but their attention is not held) and their speech is loosely associated (they pass rapidly from topic to topic).

(g) They may be openly erotic in speech or behavior.

(4) The patients remain oriented, lucid, and do not have delusions.

(5) Persons with chronic hypomania may accomplish much, although at times they may embark on schemes which either fail or which they abandon.

(6) They usually refuse to accept the fact that they are emotionally ill.

c. Acute mania

(1) These patients are obviously psychotic. They are loquacious, often incoherent, and there is a marked flight of ideas.

(2) Characteristically,

(a) They are extremely distractible and often disoriented.

(b) They tend to rhyme, pun, and make clang associations (plays on words related by sound).

(c) Psychomotor excitement is marked. Patients shout, throw things, and continually move about.

(d) They are noisy, haughty, arrogant, and demanding.

(e) They are verbally abusive, expansive, and overactive.

(f) They are sometimes sexually indecent.

(g) At times, they may become combative.

(h) Emotionally, they are aggressive, irritable, and self-exalting.

(3) Delusions of grandeur are often present (often in relationship to wealth, sexual prowess, or power).

(4) Hallucinations are also sometimes present.

(5) Paranoid traits are often evident.

d. Delirious mania

(1) Characterized by marked aggravation of the conditions described above (severe overactivity, extreme hostility, destructiveness, assaultiveness, and paranoid behavior).

(2) Since the advent of modern psychiatric treatment, including the use of somatic therapies, lithium, antidepressant agents, and neuroleptic agents, the delirious manias are rarely seen.

IX. Clinical course
   A. Depression
      1. Depressive episodes
         a. The onset is variable, with symptoms developing over a period of a few days to weeks.
         b. Many depressive episodes are self-limiting and remit without specific treatment.
         c. With treatment, the duration of episodes has been reduced from several months to a few weeks.
         d. It is estimated that at least half of the individuals with a major depressive episode will eventually have another one.
      2. Chronic depression
         a. About 15 percent of depressive disorders run a chronic course.
         b. The patients continue to experience depressed mood, sleep disturbances, and various bodily symptoms.
   B. Elations or manic episodes
      1. Most patients with manic episodes also have depressions.
      2. Before the advent of the psychotropic drugs (neuroleptic agents, antianxiety agents, lithium, and electroconvulsive therapy), the episodes were usually longer.
      3. Manic episodes are frequently recurrent.
      4. Before the introduction of lithium, only about 25 percent of manic patients had only one episode.
   C. Diagnostic categories of affective disorders
      1. Major affective disorders (major manic or depressive episodes)
         a. Bipolar disorder (manic-depressive disease)
            (1) Mixed
            (2) Manic
            (3) Depressed
         b. Major depression (psychotic depressive reaction; involutional melancholia; and some cases of depressive neurosis)
            (1) Single episode
            (2) Recurrent
      2. Other specific affective disorders
         a. Cyclothymic disorder (cyclothymic personality) includes hypomania
         b. Dysthymic disorder or, depressive neurosis (mild intermittent or sustained depression of at least two years duration)
      3. Atypical affective disorders
         a. Atypical bipolar disorder
         b. Atypical depression
X. Prevalence
   A. Depression is a very common symptom. Some estimates indicate that as many as 30 percent of people develop a depression during their lifetime.

B. At any one time, about 15 percent of the population is said to be depressed. Many, however, need never see a physician, and perhaps only a fifth or a quarter of all depressed people receive treatment.
C. Depressions occur two to four times more frequently in women than in men.
D. In the past, it was thought that manic depressive disease was a disorder of the upper-middle and the upper classes, but subsequent investigators have found no relationship between social class and bipolar affective disorders.

XI. Etiology
A. Genetic factors
1. There is an increased frequency of affective illness, particularly bipolar affective illness or disorder, in the relatives of affectively disordered patients.
2. Studies show a concordance of 68 percent for monozygotic (identical) twins in the incidence of manic depressive disease.
3. Thus, in affective disorder, there is evidence of a genetic factor.
4. Studies also support the use of a bipolar-unipolar classification.
B. Biological factors
Certain biological factors, other than genetic, seem to be important. Included are
1. Neurophysiological changes
2. Neuroendocrine abnormalities
3. Neurochemical alterations of the biogenic amines. (See biogenic amine theory under Psychopharmacology in the chapter, "Treatment in Psychiatry.")
C. Environmental stress and life events
1. Most clinical psychiatrists believe there is a relationship between the onset of depression and environmental stress. Some believe that such events play the major role.
2. Some recent research confirms a relationship between stressful environmental factors (e.g., death or losses) and the onset of depression.
D. Psychodynamic factors
1. In the past, it was believed that the dependent person with a low self-esteem and a strong superego was more prone to depression. Subsequent clinical findings have not supported the existence of a single personality type or constellation of personality traits.
2. In the past, it was assumed that hostility turned inward was important in the development of the depression. While this dynamic formulation enjoys wide clinical acceptance, research does not support it.
3. At present, the psychodynamic hypotheses are chiefly of empirical value, assisting the therapist to formulate a therapeutic program.

XII. Treatment
A. Depression

There are many effective treatments for the depressive disorders, including drugs, various psychotherapy modalities, and electroconvulsive therapy. A pluralistic approach seems indicated.

1. Drugs
   a. Antidepressant agents are used (tricyclic anti-depressants, monoamines oxidaze inhibitors).
   b. Occasionally psychomotor stimulants (amphetamine and methylphenidate) are administered.
   c. Sedatives and anti-anxiety agents are prescribed for co-existing symptoms of anxiety and tension.
   d. Neuroleptics (e.g., the phenothiazines) are useful in treating agitated people.
2. Electroconvulsive therapy
   Will relieve most depressions, although it is used less since the advent of the antidepressant agents.
3. Psychotherapy
   a. A number of treatment modalities may be used with acutely depressed patients. Most respond to some type of supportive treatment (for details, see the chapter, "Treatment in Psychiatry").
   b. Most important in the psychotherapeutic management of the acute depressive episode is that the therapist be available and active.
4. Hospitalization
   a. Most depressed patients can be treated outside of the hospital.
   b. Patients with severe depressions, suicidal urges, or medical conditions that require extensive evaluations should probably be hospitalized.
   c. With modern treatment, the average stay is three to four weeks.
5. Clinical treatment
   In clinical practice, most patients are treated with a combination of psychotherapy and medication.
6. Maintenance therapy
   For those with recurrent episodes or chronic symptoms, maintenance therapy consisting of antidepressants or other neuroleptics, as appropriate, plus supportive psychotherapy seems to be effective. Lithium is often used (see treatment of mania, below).

B. Mania
1. Persons with hypomania, or mild elations, can often be treated as outpatients.

2. Hospitalization is indicated for patients who are acutely manic. Aside from specific treatment for the episodes, patients need to be protected from the social consequences of their expansive behavior and poor judgment.
3. Medicines
   a. Lithium carbonate shortens periods of elation and helps prevent attacks of either depression or elation when administered as part of a maintenance program.
   b. Neuroleptics, especially the phenothiazines and the butyrophenones are effective in controlling the maniacal symptoms. In clinical practice, since it usually takes several days for lithium to become effective, lithium and phenothiazines, (e.g., Thorazine or Mellaril) or a butyrophenone (e.g., Haldol) are prescribed simultaneously. When the elation comes under control, the phenothiazine or butyrophenone is gradually withdrawn.
4. Occasionally, when the episode does not respond to drugs, electroconvulsive therapy is prescribed.
C. Bipolar disorders
   1. The goal is to prevent recurrences of acute episodes, relieve chronic low-grade disturbing symptoms, and improve the patient's adjustment.
   2. The most effective clinical approach seems to be combined drug therapy and psychotherapy.
   3. Medicines
      a. Lithium carbonate, other neuroleptic drugs, and supportive psychodynamic psychotherapy are often combined.
      b. Antidepressants must be administered judiciously to people who have manic episodes since it is possible to precipitate an elation in the course of long-term maintenance therapy.
   4. Occasionally, electroconvulsive therapy is used on a maintenance basis to prevent relapses. Such treatment is given at intervals of four, six, or eight weeks for several months or years. It has proved effective in some cases that have not responded to direct maintenance alone.

XIII. Case examples
A. Major depressive disorder, single episode

Mrs. S., a thirty-five-year-old housewife, was admitted to the hospital complaining of nausea, vomiting, crying, and depression. Her symptoms had begun four months earlier, following an incident that should have made her feel hostile toward her husband. However, because of guilt related to an extramarital affair a few years earlier, she was unable to express her hostile feelings and these became redirected against herself and produced the depressive symptoms.

On admission, she appeared depressed and cried rather easily when discussing her illness and her husband. There was no obvious psychomotor retardation, but she did complain of some difficulty in concentration. In the hospital, she ate poorly and had difficulty sleeping. She responded promptly to treatment and has remained free of symptoms for several years.

This patient had a single depressive episode, with symptoms common to most depressions, namely, depressed mood, difficulty in concentration, disturbance of appetite and sleep, and somatic symptoms.

B. Manic disorder, single episode

A forty-three-year-old married man was admitted to a closed psychiatric unit at the request of his family, after "uncontrolled" behavior. On admission, he was agitated, hyperactive, uncooperative, out of touch with reality, and had flight of ideas and rambling incoherent speech. He angrily ordered the nurses around. These symptoms had developed over a period of a few weeks, during which he was on strike. He first became insomniac and drank excessively.

Physical and laboratory examinations were normal. A brain scan was reported as within normal limits. He responded to treatment, including lithium and Haldol.

He had never had any previous affective symptoms. His family history revealed one sister who has had schizophrenic disorder.

It was not clear whether his excessive alcoholic intake was causal or symptomatic of the manic episode. At any rate, this seems to be an example of a single manic episode.

C. Bipolar disorder

Mr. S., a forty-one-year-old attorney, was admitted to the hospital in an acute manic episode. He was extremely hyperactive, distractible, irritable, and demanding. He had a marked flight of ideas and expressed hostility toward his wife for what he described an infidelity. Eight years earlier, he had developed a depressive episode following his wife's severe infectious disease, and since that time he had developed manic symptoms every spring and depressive symptoms every fall. Prior to the onset of his illness, he was described as perfectionistic, egotistical, and outgoing. Between episodes, he practiced law with above-average skill and showed no evidence of personality deterioration.

This is a classical case of manic-depressive illness. The patient's behavior on admission—elated mood, flight of ideas, and increased activity—was typical of acute mania. Note, also, the absence of personality deterioration between attacks.

D. Major depressive disorder, recurrent

Mr. N., a fifty-five-year-old accountant, was admitted to the hospital with a severe depression which had begun following the accidental injury of his son nine months earlier. He showed marked psychomotor retardation, refused to eat, and was mute most of the time. When he did speak, he expressed delusions of worthlessness, hopelessness, and nihilism. His history revealed three previous episodes of depression, beginning at age twenty. Only the first attack had been severe enough to require hospital treatment. During the other episodes, he was able to work, but with reduced efficiency. He was described as a quiet, shy, conscientious, sensitive person who worried unduly about his work and family.

This is a case of major depressive disorder characterized by several episodes of depression and an absence of personality deterioration between attacks. The marked psychomotor retardation, the muteness, the refusal to eat, and the delusions characterize the last attack as a stuporous depression.

E. Other examples of bipolar disorder
   1. John Ruskin (1819–1900) writer, critic, artist and author of *Modern Painters* was an example of a bipolar disorder, swinging from elation to misery, always sensitive and always expressive.
   2. Vincent W. Van Gogh (1853–1890), Dutch painter, suffered from mood swings, alternating between profound depression and extreme exuberance. On Christmas Eve, 1888, he cut off part of his left ear and in July 1890, he committed suicide.

XIV. Involutional melancholia
A. Definition
   1. The term *involutional melancholia* was used to describe a psychotic reaction with initial onset in the involutional period (late middle life), most commonly characterized by depressive affect but occasionally by paranoid mentation.
   2. This diagnostic category has been dropped in *DSM*-III. Cases previously diagnosed as involutional depression would probably now be described as "major depressive disorder."
   3. The disorder is also known as *involutional depression.*
B. Prevalence
   Despite the fact that life expectancy has steadily increased, the frequency of cases has greatly decreased. It has probably become less common because patients who develop signs of depression are treated promptly and classic involutional depression seldom develops.
C. Case example

Mr. J., a sixty-five-year-old man, was admitted to the hospital complaining of loss of appetite, insomnia, weight loss, depression, and constipation. His illness began six months earlier when he was retired from his job as a shop foreman. He had always enjoyed good physical health and had never had an emotional illness. He had no interests aside from his work, and was described by his family as serious, conscientious, rigid, and hardworking.

On admission, he was obviously depressed and cried frequently. He showed psychomotor retardation, complained of difficulty in thinking, and was preoccupied with his constipation, believing that his bowels had dried up because he had no bowel movements. He was self-deprecatory and at times did not wish to eat because he thought he was unworthy. Treated with electroconvulsive therapy, he made an excellent recovery and remained well for several years.

The onset of a delusional depression in the involutional period would have characterized this disorder as an involutional depressive reaction in the past. At present, it would be diagnosed as a major depressive disorder.

References

American Psychiatric Association. *Diagnostic and Statistical Manual.* 3d ed. Washington, D. C.: 1978–1979.

Eaton, M. T., Jr.; Peterson, M. H.; and David, J. A. *Psychiatry.* 3d ed. Flushing, N. Y.: Medical Examination Publishing Company, 1976, chaps. 9, 10, 11.

Freedman, A. M.; Kaplan, H. I.; and Sadock, B. J. *Modern Synopsis of Comprehensive Textbook of Psychiatry.* Vol. 2. Baltimore: Williams & Wilkins Company, 1976, chaps. 16, 17, 28.

Goodwin, D. W., and Guze, S. B. *Psychiatric Diagnosis.* 2d ed. New York: Oxford University Press, 1979, chap. 1.

Kolb, L. C. *Modern Clinical Psychiatry.* 9th ed. Philadelphia: W. B. Saunders Company, 1977, chap. 20.

Nicholi, A. M., Jr., ed. *The Harvard Guide to Modern Psychiatry.* Cambridge: Belknap Press of Harvard University, 1978, chaps. 13, 28.

Robbins, E., et al. "Primary and Secondary Affective Disorders." In J. Zubin and F. A. Frehan (Eds.), *Disorders of Mood.* Baltimore: John Hopkins University Press, 1974, chap. 1.

Schneidman, E. S. "Suicide." In A. M. Freedman; N. I. Kaplan; and B. J. Sadock (Eds.), *Comprehensive Textbook of Psychiatry,* vol 2, 2d ed. Baltimore: The Williams & Wilkins Company, 1976.

Scheidman, E. S., and Faberow, N. L. *A Cry for Help.* New York: McGraw-Hill Book Company, 1961.

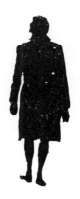

We are prone to the malady of the introvert, who, with the manifold spectacle of the world spread out before him, turns away and gazes only upon the emptiness within. But, let us not imagine that there is anything grand about the introvert's unhappiness.

Bertrand Russell: *The Conquest of Happiness* **(1930)**

Schizophrenic Disorders

I. Historical notes

A. The syndromes that are now classified as schizophrenia have been recognized for at least 3,400 years, although in the past they have carried varying labels.

B. Greek physicians in the 5th century B.C. termed it *dementia* and distinguished it from mania and melancholia.

C. Benedict Augustin Morel (1860) introduced the term *demence precoce* to describe psychosis in a fourteen-year-old boy.

D. E. Hecker (1871) described *hebephrenia* as a progressive psychotic illness of rapid onset in adolescence.

E. K. Kahlbaum (1874) described *catatonia, or tension insanity,* and assumed it to be a symptom of some organic brain disease. His description was of a condition characterized by muteness, immobility, waxy flexibility, and so forth.

F. Emil Kraepelin (1896), believing that all of the above syndromes were related, classified them into one group called *dementia praecox.*

G. Adolph Meyer (1906) theorized that dementia praecox is a type of reaction (*parergastic reaction*).

H. Eugen Bleuler (1911) coined the term *schizophrenia* to emphasize the "splitting" of the personality (from the Greek *schizo,* "to split"; and *phren,* "mind").

I. Jacob Kasan (1933) described *schizoaffective psychosis.*

J. G. Langfeldt (1949) described *reactive schizophrenia,* or *schizophreniform psychosis.*

K. Paul Hoch and P. Polatin (1949) described *pseudoneurotic schizophrenia.*

II. Definition

"A large group of disorders, usually of psychotic proportion, manifested by characteristic disturbances of language and communication, thought, perception, affect, and behavior which last longer than six months. Thought disturbances are marked by alterations of concept formation that may lead to misinterpretation of reality, misperceptions, and sometimes delusions and hallucinations."[1]

III. Prevalence

A. Schizophrenia occurs in less than 1 percent of the population.

B. The incidence of schizophreniform disorders, (see section, Schizophrenic-like disorders) is unknown, but the combined prevalence of the two disorders is probably somewhere between 1 and 2 percent.

C. Although schizophrenic disorders affect a small percentage of the population, patients with these disorders occupy a significant proportion of mental hospital beds.

---

1. Definition from *A Psychiatric Glossary,* 5th ed., American Psychiatric Association, Washington, D.C., 1980.

D. According to Freedman et al., somewhere between 460,000 to 940,000 people will need treatment annually for this disorder.

E. It is most prevalent between the ages of fifteen and fifty-four.

F. An estimated two million Americans suffer from schizophrenia.

IV. Conceptions of schizophrenia

A. Emil Kraepelin believed that dementia praecox resulted from injury to the germ plasm or from some metabolic disorder which caused autointoxication. Thus, he thought of it as an organically caused disease. He was the first to include hebephrenic, catatonic, and paranoid reactions under one category.

B. Eugen Bleuler's concept was broader than Kraepelin's. Although he believed this illness to be primarily of physical origin, he did consider certain secondary symptoms (such as delusions, hallucinations, and mannerisms) to be psychogenic (an indicative attempt at adaptation to the primary disturbance). He emphasized the "splitting of the various mental functions" (i.e., the coexistence of disharmonious complexes). He regarded the formal mechanism underlying schizophrenic symptoms as the loosening of association.

C. Adolph Meyer regarded this as a maladaptive reaction ("the accumulation of life-long faulty habits of adaptation in the setting of an inferior psychobiological endowment"). That is, he saw it as a habit disorganization. He emphasized longitudinal (versus cross-sectional) psychological factors.

D. Sigmund Freud regarded schizophrenia as withdrawal and regression associated with a weak ego, a return to early narcissism (i.e., the libido is withdrawn from external objects and directed toward the ego).

E. Carl Jung believed that schizophrenia arises when the psyche is unable to rid itself of a complex and can no longer adapt to the surroundings. Thus, separation from reality results. He thought that delusions, hallucinations, and other schizophrenic symptoms were due to an autochthonous complex (i.e., a group of ideas which, because they were disturbing, were removed from consciousness and maintained in an independent existence).

F. Harry Stack Sullivan regarded schizophrenia as the indirect outcome of unhealthy interpersonal relationships between the child (who later becomes schizophrenic) and the parents.

G. The double-bind theory

In 1960, Bateson hypothesized a "double bind" to account for schizophrenia. He theorized that learning occurs in a context with formal characteristics and that this context exists within a broader context, a "metacontext." Occurrences in the narrow context are affected by the metacontext. There may be conflict or discordance between the metacontext and the context; for example, learning in a context set within a primitive metacontext would produce discordance. Thus, Bateson explains, the individual is confronted with the dilemma of "being wrong in the primary context or being right for the wrong reasons or in the wrong way. This is the so-called double bind." Whether such a double bind is unique to schizophrenic patients is not really known at this time. According to Kolb:

> the schizophrenic may be seen as fixed in an intense, emotional relationship with a parent who, by the contradictions between her verbal remarks and behavior, makes it impossible for the former to discriminate properly or to respond for clarification, as his questioning is treated as a threat to the needed relationship by the parent. A concrete example is a schizophrenic adolescent who, tied to his mother verbally, is encouraged to use initiative in his schoolwork, yet when he attempts to leave home to visit the library, he is told he must not do so as the parent needs him and will become ill in his absence. Such a double bind restricts and confuses the development of clear communications, since the parent's position is inconsistent, and also limits the son's healthful socialization with others, from which he might learn progressive social discriminations and develop the potentiality for evolving other healthy relations.
>
> Whether the double bind is characteristic of schizophrenic families alone or has special features for such families is not known.[2]

   H. Silvano Arieti regards schizophrenia as a reaction to an extremely severe state of anxiety originating in childhood and reactivated later in life. It occurs when no other possibility of adjustment is available to the patient.

   I. Family psychopathology

     Studies in this area have been made from two points of view—

      1. Research concerned with psychodynamic interaction between individuals.

      2. Socially oriented research that seems concerned with the individual's reaction to psychopathology within the family. Most of the studies have been concerned with psychopathology in the parental family, although some have been concerned with the psychopathology in the marital family.

   J. Phenomenological-existential concepts

      1. Binswanger is the best known exponent. His case reports are concerned with the underlying structure that existed prior to the illness.

V. Etiology

   A. The cause of schizophrenia is unknown.

      1. Conflicting findings by different investigators lead to the belief that schizophrenia is really several different disorders.

---

2. From: Kolb, L. E. *Modern Clinical Psychiatry,* 9th ed. Philadelphia: W. B. Saunders Company, 1977.

2. Others describe two major types: (1) "process," which does not respond to treatment, has a poor prognosis, and is probably biologically determined; and (2) "reactive," a remitting type that has a more favorable prognosis and is probably related to experiential factors.

B. Theories of etiology can be divided into
   1. Biological
   2. Sociocultural
   3. Experiential, or psychological

C. Biological theories include
   1. Genetic predisposition
      a. Some studies suggest a genetic factor in schizophrenic disorders. However, many authorities who believe that there is some genetic predisposition also believe that subsequent factors (biological, psychological, social, or experiential), are necessary for the production of a schizophrenic disorder.
      b. Studies indicate that children of schizophrenic parents are much more likely to develop the disorder than the general population. The expectancy of schizophrenia in children of one schizophrenic parent is 16 percent versus 0.85 percent for the general population. In families where both parents are schizophrenic, the expectancy in the children is 40 percent.
      c. Kalmann's studies of twins also suggest a genetic factor.
         (1) Among monozygotic (identical) twins, if one is schizophrenic, 85 percent of the other twins will also be.
         (2) Among dizygotic (fraternal) twins, the correlation is 14 percent, about the same as among other siblings.
      d. On the basis of presently available information, we cannot label schizophrenia an hereditary disease, but it does seem that an hereditary predisposition is present in many, if not all, cases.
   2. Biochemical predisposition
      a. There has been a remarkable increase in our knowledge of brain biochemistry and psychopharmacology in recent years.
      b. Transmethylation hypothesis
         Harley-Mason theorized that, since many hallucinogens are methylated substances, an accumulation of methylated substances might occur in schizophrenia. Methylated indoleamine has been found in the blood and urine of schizophrenics.

c. Dopamine hypothesis
    (1) Schizophrenia is assumed to reflect a defect in dopamine-mediated brain systems.
    (2) Amphetamines, which stimulate release of catecholamines, can also produce psychotic symptoms that resemble schizophrenia and exacerbate psychotic symptoms of acute schizophrenia.
    (3) The class of antipsychotics (phenothiazines) most effective in treating schizophrenic symptoms, acts to inhibit or block dopamine-mediated transmissions.
d. Whether the reported findings of neurohumoral transmission are of primary etiological significance in the production of schizophrenia or whether they represent a "final common biochemical pathway" is not known.

D. Sociocultural theories
  1. There is a high density of schizophrenics in urban ghettos and other underprivileged areas of the city. This finding has led to two contradictory theories.
    a. The "downward-drift" theory states that schizophrenics drift to such areas because they are socially and economically incompetent.
    b. These areas "breed" schizophrenics because they are populated by people laden with severe socioeconomic problems. In other words, the schizophrenic has never experienced achievement.
  2. Social and economic limitations prevent the achievement of fundamental gratification.
  3. There is a higher incidence of broken homes in the lower socioeconomic areas.

E. Experiential, or psychological, theory
  1. Psychoanalytic theories
    a. Freud emphasized the role of sexual regression in the development of the illness.
    b. Melanie Klein emphasized the importance of early mother-child relationships.
    c. Harry Stack Sullivan emphasized the patient's deeply disturbed interpersonal relationships, rather than the intrapsychic mechanisms emphasized by Freud and Klein.
    d. Gregory Bateson suggested that repeated exposure to double-bind experiences makes the potential schizophrenic perceive the entire environment as a double bind.

F. Multiple causation
    1. A review of the above theories and findings suggests that there are multiple causative factors operating in the production of schizophrenia.

VI. Psychopathology
  A. Most psychiatrists regard schizophrenic disorder as regression (see the Freudian concept, above, and the section on regression in the chapter, "Adaptations to Anxiety").
    1. There is withdrawal of interest from the environment and loss of interest in objects and other persons.
    2. According to psychoanalytic theory, this is regression to a level at which schizophrenics, like infants, are incapable of distinguishing themselves from the environment (i.e., regression to primary narcissism).
  B. Those having paranoid delusions are also overusing the mechanism of projection (see "Adaptations to Anxiety").
  C. The prepsychotic personality is often schizoid (introverted), schizotypal, or borderline.
  D. Precipitating factors may or may not be evident, and their effect varies with the individual's vulnerability. They are evident in the so called reactive types of schizophrenia.
  E. The onset may be gradual, occurring in the absence of obvious precipitating factors, as in so-called process schizophrenia.

VII. Symptomatology
  A. Since our present-day concept of this disorder includes varying clinical types, it is difficult to present a "typical" cluster of symptoms.
  B. Bleuler
    1. Bleuler described four main symptoms: (a) disturbance of association; (b) disturbance of affect; (c) autism; and (d) heightened ambivalence. These are often called the "four A's."
      a. Disburbance of association is looseness of association. It is called *derailment* in the *Diagnostic and Statistical Manual of Mental Disorders,* 3d ed. (*DSM*-III). In schizophrenic speech, successive ideas appear to be unrelated or only slightly related to each other.
      b. Disturbances of affect usually take the form of flatness, bluntness, or inappropriateness.
      c. Autism is fantasy and day-dreaming that substitutes for reality.
      d. Heightened ambivalence is exaggeration of co-existing opposite feelings or emotions for the same person, thing, situation, or goal.

2. In addition, Bleuler believed that the main accessory or secondary symptoms need to be present. In severe or advanced cases they are usually found. They are: (a) delusions; (b) hallucinations; and (c) ideas of reference. Ideas of reference include feelings of thought control and feelings of influence.

C. According to *DSM*-III, the essential features of this group of disorders are:

1. Disorganization of previous level of functioning. Significant impairment occurs in the areas of routine daily functioning, such as occupation, socialization, and self-care.

2. Presence of certain psychotic features during the active phase of the illness.

3. Characteristic symptoms involving multiple psychological processes.

   a. Disturbance of language and communication

   Incoherence is a common symptom; neologistic speech is rarer. Common communication disorders in schizophrenic are derailment (loosening of associations), poverty of content of speech, and illogicality.

   (1) Poverty of speech content means overly concrete, repetitive, or stereotyped speech. Little if any information has been conveyed, although the individual has spoken at some length.

   (2) Illogicality means that facts are obscured, distorted, or excluded, and that conclusions are based on inadequate or faulty evidence.

   (3) Perseveration and blocking are less common communication disorders.

   b. Major disturbances

   Delusions may be persecutory, referential, or of thought broadcasting (the belief that thoughts are broadcast from the schizophrenic's head to the external world).

   (1) Thought insertion is the delusion that thoughts that are not the patients' own are inserted into their minds.

   (2) Thought withdrawal is the delusion that thoughts have been removed from their heads.

   (3) Other delusions are of being controlled or of passivity (feelings, impulses, thoughts, or actions are not their own and are imposed on them by some external force).

   (4) Somatic, grandiose, religious, and nihilistic delusions are less common.

c. Disturbances of perception
   (1) The major perceptual distortions are hallucinations.
   (2) Although they may involve any of the senses directly, by far the most common are auditory hallucinations.
d. Disturbances of affect
   (1) Blunting, flattening, or inappropriateness.
   (2) Anti-psychotic drugs can produce a state that is similar to flattening.
e. Disturbances of the sense of self
   (1) Also referred to as *loss of ego boundaries*.
   (2) They may manifest themselves as morbid perplexity about one's identity and the meaning of existence, or in some of the specific delusions described above, particularly those involving control by some outside forces.
f. Disturbances of volition
   (1) Inadequate interest, drive, or ability to complete a course of action.
   (2) Anti-psychotic medications may produce akinesia or sedation, which resemble volitional disturbance.
g. Disturbances of relationship to the external world
   (1) Frequently, there is withdrawal and a preoccupation with ideas and fantasies that are egocentric and illogical.
   (2) Severe forms are referred to as *autism*.
h. Disturbances of motor behavior
   (1) There may be marked decrease in reactivity to the environment, most marked in catatonic stupor.
   (2) Patients may maintain a rigid posture and resist efforts to move them, as in catatonic rigidity.
   (3) There may be stereotyped excited motor behavior, as in catatonic excitement.
   (4) The patients may voluntarily assume inappropriate or bizarre postures, as in catatonic posturing.
   (5) They may resist and actively counteract instructions or attempts to move them, as in catatonic negativism.
   (6) In addition, there may be mannerisms, grimacing, or waxy flexibility.
i. Associated features
   Any number of other psychiatric symptoms may occur. These include—
   (1) Perplexed, disheveled or eccentric appearance.

(2) Dysphoric mood.

(3) Depersonalization, derealization, simple ideas of reference, and illusions are common.

VIII. Clinical types

Because of the varied clinical picture, cases are classified into different clinical types depending upon the predominant symptomatology. In *DSM*-III, the following phenomenological subtypes are described:

A. Disorganized type

Also called *hebephrenic,* after Hebe, the Greek goddess of youth.

1. The essential features are marked incoherence and flat, incongruous, or silly affect; absence of systematized delusions; and frequent incoherence.

2. Associated features include grimacing, mannerisms, hypochondriacal complaints, extreme social withdrawal, and other oddities of behavior.

3. There is usually an early and insidious onset.

4. The course is usually chronic, and without remissions.

5. Case example.

Mary, a twenty-one-year-old stenographer, was brought to the hospital by the police who had been called after she had entered a strange residence at 1:00 A.M. in response to an uncontrollable urge to urinate. She had always been a shy, introverted, and intensely religious girl. Three years earlier, after high school graduation, she had had a "nervous breakdown" that required six months' hospitalization. She showed improvement following that treatment, but still seemed shy and self-contained, and behaved inappropriately at times.

Three days before her second admission to the hospital she became restless, sleepless, and spent the night on her knees in continuous prayer. The following morning she seemed elated and became upset by several commonplace incidents. She started out for work, but in response to "voices" went instead to religious services at a nearby church. The second night was likewise spent in continuous prayer. The following morning, she again started out for work but became confused and returned home. The evening preceding admission, she boarded a bus to attend church but became confused "because my friend Anne prayed that I would get mixed up" and left the bus far from church. She wandered about aimlessly, finally entering the strange residence at 1:00 A.M.

On admission she was obviously disturbed. She was preoccupied with religious and moral ideas and said that God was talking to her through the newspapers, radio, and television. She repeatedly misidentified the ward personnel as apostles, disciples, and other biblical characters. Her affect was euphoric and inappropriate. She was physically active, making frequent changes in posture and moving about the room aimlessly. She was unkempt and continuously disrobed.

Despite a three-month stay in the hospital, during which time she received thirty electroconvulsive treatments, there was no sustained improvement in her behavior and she was committed to a state hospital for prolonged care.

In this case, note the schizoid premorbid personality, the rather definite onset of psychotic symptoms in adolescence, the obvious emotional disturbance at the time of admission, the bizarre nature of her symptoms, and her bizarre delusions and hallucinations.

B. Catatonic types
  1. Four different types of catatonic symptomatology are described in *DSM*-III.
    a. Catatonic stupor or mutism
      Characterized by mutism, markedly decreased reactivity to the environment, reduction of spontaneous movements and activities.
    b. Catatonic rigidity
      Patients maintain a rigid posture against efforts to move them.
    c. Catatonic excitement
      Characterized by extreme psychomotor agitation, purposeless and stereotyped excited motor activity not influenced by external stimuli. Such a patient seems motivated from within and is often dangerous.
    d. Catatonic posturing
      Voluntary assumption of inappropriate or bizarre posture.
  2. Onset and course
    The onset of catatonic schizophrenia is usually sudden, and the course is usually short.
  3. Prognosis
    Good for recovery from the episode, but guarded about future recurrences.
  4. Case example, catatonic stupor

  Miss J., a thirty-nine-year-old secretary, was brought to the hospital by her two sisters because her behavior had been bizarre for a week. She was described as a quiet, reserved person who had few friends and preferred to remain by herself. Although she danced occasionally, she was generally shy in the company of men. She had no symptoms of emotional illness until seven days earlier, when she suddenly began to abstain from food. Five days later she expressed religious delusions, became self-condemnatory, refused to go to bed at night, and demanded to see a priest at 3:00 A.M. A few hours later, she was admitted to a general hospital and given intravenous feedings because of her refusal to eat. She would not remain in bed and left the hospital against advice. At home she continued to refuse food. Finally, her sisters sought her admission to the hospital.

  On admission she was negativistic, refusing food, medication, and nursing care. She was mute most of the time, and when she did speak she expressed religious delusions and hallucinations. She postured, that is, assumed uncomfortable postures for long periods, and exhibited waxy flexibility, that is, her extremities would remain in positions in which they were placed.

She recovered from this episode after a course of electroconvulsive therapy and was discharged to her home at the end of one month. A few weeks later, the symptoms recurred. This second episode also responded rather promptly to treatment, and she was discharged after six weeks. She has remained well for several years.

The characteristic features in the foregoing case of catatonic stupor are the sudden onset of negativism, mutism, posturizing, and waxy flexibility; the good response to treatment in both instances; and the prepsychotic schizoid personality.

5. Case example, catatonic excitement

P. H., a twenty-year-old college student, was brought to the hospital in restraints by the police. His illness had become manifest the previous day, when he began expressing delusions of grandeur and persecution. He left his fraternity house without telling anyone where he was going and remained away all night. About two hours before admission, the police were summoned to pick him up in a nearby suburb because of bizarre behavior characterized by agitation, assaultiveness, and disrobing. Before the onset of his illness he was described as conscientious, compulsive, and meek. He resisted accepting responsibility and had an "inferiority complex."

On admission he was uncooperative, mute, belligerent, agitated, and assaultive. He refused food, medications, and nursing care, and was careless of his excreta. After a series of electroconvulsive treatment, he became cooperative and calm. Treatment was continued in another hospital to which he was transferred in order to be nearer his parents.

Mutism, negativism, agitation, assaultiveness, and violent behavior characterized this case as catatonic excitement.

6. Periodic catatonic type
This is a rare form of episodic catatonia that is related to shifts in the individual's metabolic nitrogen balance. Maintenance on neuroleptic drugs prevents recurrence.

C. Paranoid type
1. Essential features
a. A clinical picture that is dominated by the relative persistence of or preoccupation with delusions that are usually persecutory but may be grandiose in nature; or by hallucinations with a persecutory or grandiose content.

b. In addition, there may be delusions of jealousy.

2. Associated features
Anger, argumentativeness, violence, fearfulness, delusions of reference, and concerns about autonomy, gender identity, and sexual preference.

3. Onset

Often abrupt and usually occurs in adult life, later than the other subtypes.

4. Case example

> Mrs. L., a thirty-year-old housewife, was brought to the hospital by her family because she had behaved strangely for the preceding seven months. The behavior was characterized by withdrawal, inappropriate mood, preoccupation with religious ideas, and delusions that her husband and the family physician were "trying to poison the food." In preschool years she had been overly attached to her mother, but she subsequently became so interested in outdoor activities that she was considered a tomboy.
>
> In the hospital, she was markedly suspicious of the entire staff, accusing them of poisoning her food, talking about her, gambling, and so forth. She said she received messages from Christ, whose voice came to her over the radio. Much of the time she was withdrawn, but at times she talked readily though inappropriately. Her affect was flattened.
>
> Following a course of electroconvulsive therapy, she improved, and returned home. Eighteen months later, the same symptoms recurred and she was readmitted to the hospital. Though the second episode was more refractory to treatment, she did improve sufficiently to return home after eight months.

D. Undifferentiated types

This category is characterized by

1. Prominent psychotic symptoms that cannot be classified in any of the other categories, or
2. Characteristics of more than one clinical subtype.

E. Residual types

1. This category is for those individuals who have had an episode of schizophrenic illness, whose current clinical picture does not contain any prominent psychotic symptoms, but in whom some signs of the disorder persist.
2. This is equivalent of the category, *in partial remission.*
3. Examples of persistent symptoms are emotional blunting, social withdrawal, eccentric behavior, and persistent but inconspicuous delusions or hallucinations.

IX. Cultural influences

A. Records suggest that the incidence of schizophrenia in this country has probably remained essentially unchanged during the past century, perhaps even longer.
B. Cultural factors, however, have had an influence on the relative frequency and character of schizophrenic symptoms.
C. Simple schizophrenia is rarely, if ever, diagnosed anymore. In *DSM*-III, such cases are probably classified as schizoid personality or schizotypal personality.

D. Catatonic forms of schizophrenia seem less frequent.

E. Schizophrenics are less aggressive than they were a quarter of a century ago, perhaps in part because of the early prescription of antipsychotic medications that reduce assaultive and antisocial behavior.

F. Although paranoid reactions have increased, delusions of grandeur, witchcraft, and other magic have become less frequent, whereas ideas of being hypnotized or influenced by electronics or radiation have increased.

G. The content of delusions has become more realistic and plausible.

X. Course and prognosis

A. Schizophrenia was once regarded as a progressive disorder with a poor or hopeless prognosis.

B. As can be noted from the *DSM*-III classification, episodic types of the disorder are now recognized. These are many times followed by symptom-free periods, long periods of remission. Occasionally, individuals have been observed to have a single mild schizophrenic or (schizophrenic-like) attack, without any recurrence.

C. As noted earlier, schizophrenic disorders can occur either in attacks or as a progressive disease; thus, we speak of "reactive" and "process" schizophrenic disorder.

D. However, it still must be regarded as a tenacious disorder.

E. Currently, there is more optimism about arrest and recovery in this illness, chiefly because of the favorable effect of psychotropic drugs.

F. In general, however, the prognosis is guarded.

G. Certain criteria have become more or less accepted for prognosticating the outcome of any case of schizophrenic disorder.
   1. The following are considered favorable prognostic signs:
      a. Sudden or acute onset
      b. Conspicuous precipitating factors
      c. Catatonic symptoms
      d. The presence of affective symptoms, i.e., depression or elation; perhaps these cases are more properly classified as schizoaffective disorders in the present nomenclature
      e. The presence of confusion
      f. The history of a good previous social adjustment
      g. Married schizophrenics have a better outlook than single, divorced, or widowed ones
      h. Stable employment (the schizophrenic has a job to which to return)
      i. Cooperativeness (the patient cooperates with the treatment regime)
      j. An empathic therapist.

2. The following are considered unfavorable signs:
   a. History of previous episodes
   b. Schizoid or schizotypal premorbid personality
   c. Absence of conspicuous precipitating factors
   d. Family history of mental illness
   e. Persistence of the symptoms for more than one year
   f. The presence of sustained emotional withdrawal, aloofness, and shallow or inappropriate affect, which makes the patient less cooperative about taking maintenance medication
   g. Onset in childhood or early puberty (recovery is unlikely).

XI. Schizophrenic-like disorders
   A. Schizoaffective disorders
      1. This disorder has been defined in many different ways since it was first classified.
      2. In *A Psychiatric Glossary, schizoaffective disorder* is defined as "a depressive or manic *syndrome* that precedes or develops concurrently with *psychotic* symptoms incompatible with an affective disorder. Includes some *symptoms* characteristic or *schizophrenia* and other symptoms seen in *major affective disorders.*[3]
      3. It is usually applied to those psychotic reactions in which affective symptoms (either depressions or elations) are associated with psychotic symptoms.
      4. In *DSM*-III, this category is retained without diagnostic criteria for those cases in which the clinician is unable to make a differential diagnosis between affective disorder and either schizophreniform disorder or schizophrenia, with any degree of certainty.
      5. Essentially, the symptoms of this disorder are the same as those for schizophrenia plus the affective symptoms.
      6. Schizoaffective disorders are listed separately in *DSM*-III because accumulating evidence suggests
         a. Persons with a mixture of affective and schizophrenic symptomatology have a better prognosis.
         b. The onset and resolution tend to be abrupt.
         c. The patients are more likely to recover premorbid level and function.
         d. There is usually an absence of family history, although there is an increased prevalence of affective disorders among the family members.

3. Definition from *A Psychiatric Glossary,* 5th ed., American Psychiatric Association, Washington, D.C., 1980.

B. Schizophreniform disorder
   1. In the past, the term *schizophreniform* disorders has included cases that would be now described as schizoaffective.
   2. The essential features are identical to those of schizophrenia, with the exception that the duration is less than six months but more than one week.
   3. It is classified separately because accumulated evidence suggests that it may have different correlates (i.e., emotional turmoil and confusion; a better prognosis; a tendency toward acute onset and resolution; more likely recovery to premorbid level of functioning; and absence of an increase in the prevalence of schizophrenia among the family members).
C. Brief reactive psychosis
   1. The essential feature is a psychotic disorder of at least a few hours' duration but lasting no more than one week, with a sudden onset immediately following a recognizable stressor that would be expected to evoke significant symptoms of distress in almost all individuals, for example, loss of a loved one or the psychological trauma of combat (*DSM*-III).
   2. Associated features are emotional turmoil and one of the following:
      a. Incoherence, derailment, or marked illogical thinking
      b. Delusions
      c. Hallucinations
      d. Behavior that is grossly disorganized or catatonic
   3. Predisposing factors
      a. Individuals with histrionic, schizotypal, and borderline personalities are thought to be particularly vulnerable to the development of this disorder.
      b. Alcohol or drug abuse may be factors.
      c. Situations involving catastrophic stress, such as warfare, are predisposing factors by definition.

XII. **Treatment of schizophrenia**
A. Since the etiology is incompletely understood, the treatment has been largely empirical.
B. The type of treatment depends upon the type and severity of the disorder. It can be divided into
   1. Milieu therapy
   2. Various psychotherapies (psychoanalytic, supportive, and behavioral)
   3. Somatic (electroconvulsive therapy)
   4. Chemotherapy (antipsychotic drugs)
C. Milieu therapy
The exact plan varies according to the individual needs of the patient. Included are

1. Various inpatient hospital programs.
   Although some schizophrenics can make a marginal adjustment extramurally, hospitalization is frequently indicated, at least for a period of time.
2. Various outpatient arrangements, individually arranged. These include
   a. Various living arrangements, such as halfway houses, apartments, board-and-care facilities, foster homes, and family care.
   b. Vocational arrangements, such as sheltered workshops, day activity centers, and vocational rehabilitation placements.
3. Psychological treatment
   a. Psychoanalytic psychotherapy (see section in the chapter, "Treatment in Psychiatry").
   b. In general, therapists should be active and positive in their approach.
   c. Establishing a relationship may be difficult because of the schizophrenics's distrust and inability to become close.
   d. Behavioral therapy is mostly based on the operant conditioning of B. F. Skinner. The value of this kind of treatment has yet to be determined, and should be regarded as in the experimental stage.
   e. Supportive therapy
4. Somatic therapy (electroconvulsive therapy)
   Its status is uncertain, although it has been successfully used in two types of cases, those that have not responded to drugs and acute attacks.
5. Psychosurgery is a rare form of treatment (see the chapter, "Treatment in Psychiatry").
6. Megavitamin therapy
   This treatment involves the administration of large doses of niacin. Major controlled studies indicate that niacin is no better than a placebo.
7. Chemotherapy (antipsychotic agents)
   a. Intramuscular injections of long-acting phenothiazines (such as Prolixin) may be necessary until the patient becomes cooperative.
   b. It should be kept in mind, however, that a large percentage (two-thirds or more) of schizophrenics do not comply with the drug regime after discharge.
8. Maintenance therapy may be necessary.
   a. In many cases, drugs can eventually be discontinued.
   b. However, a significant number of patients relapse when antipsychotic agents are withdrawn.

9. Combined psychotherapy and drug therapy
   Antipsychotic drugs plus "the therapeutic alliance" seems helpful to most schizophrenics.
10. The most effective treatment program is usually one combining psychotropic, psychological, and milieu therapy.
11. Results of treatment
    a. About one-third of the patients will do relatively well.
    b. One-third will become hard-core failures.
    c. The remainder will occupy an intermittent status.

References

American Psychiatric Association. *Diagnostic and Statistical Manual of Mental Disorders.* 3d ed. Washington, D. C., 1978–1979.

———. *A Psychiatric Glossary.* 4th ed. Washington, D. C., 1975.

Arieti, S. *Interpretation of Schizophrenia.* New York: Basic Books, Inc. Publishers, 1975.

Bateson, G. *Minimal Requirements for a Theory of Schizophrenia. Archives of General Psychiatry,* 1960, 2: 477.

Bleuler, E. *Dementia Praecox or the Group of Schizophrenias.* New York: International Universities Press, 1950.

Freedman, A. M.; Kaplan, H. I.; and Sadock, B. J. *Modern Synopsis of Comprehensive Textbook of Psychiatry.* Vol. 2. Baltimore: William & Wilkins Company, 1976, chap. 14.

Goodwin, D. W., and Guze, S. V. *Psychiatric Diagnosis.* 2d ed. New York: Oxford University Press, 1979, chap. 2.

Kallman. F. J. *Heredity and Health and Mental Disorder.* New York: W. W. Norton & Company, Inc., 1953.

Kolb, L. C. *Modern Clinical Psychiatry.* Philadelphia: W. B. Saunders Company, 1977, chap. 19.

Nicholi, A. M. *The Harvard Guide to Modern Psychiatry.* Cambridge: Belknap Press of Harvard University, 1978, chap. 11.

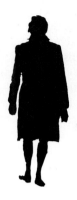

What is madness: To have
erroneous perceptions and to reason
correctly from them.

Paranoid Disorders

Voltaire: "Madness," in
Philosophical Dictionary **(1764)**

I. Definition

A. Psychotic disorders in which the predominant symptoms are delusions, generally persecutory, jealous, or grandiose. They are usually without hallucinations and cannot be explained by other psychotic disorders in which paranoid symptoms may be prominent (such as schizophrenic disorders, schizophreniform disorders, brief reactive psychosis, or organic mental disorders).

B. The paranoid disorders include
1. Paranoia (duration at least six months)
2. Acute paranoid disorder (duration less than six months)
3. Atypical paranoid disorder (paranoid state)
4. Shared paranoid disorders (*folie à deux*)

C. There are other psychotic disorders in which there are paranoid delusions, such as paranoid schizophrenia or organic delusional syndrome. For example, in paranoid psychosis, which can be caused by a chronic amphetamine toxicity, there are auditory hallucinations and stereotyped behavior, with little delirium or confusion. Such disorders are more properly classified elsewhere.

II. Introduction

A. All the paranoid disorders are characterized by overuse of the mechanism of projection (see the chapter, "Adaptations to Anxiety").

B. Although overuse of projection is pathological, it is a defense mechanism that is fairly commonly employed. For example, we blame others for our own mistakes, we may blame social ills on minority groups, militant groups such as antivivisectionists and antiflouridationists may overuse the mechanism of projection, most of us are usually critical of our own shortcomings when we find them in others.

C. Through projection, inner unconscious feelings become more acceptable in their externalized conscious form.

D. Delusions of grandeur require rationalization in addition to projection ("I'm being persecuted because I am somebody very special").

E. People with paranoid conditions are characterized by hyperalertness, oversuspiciousness, distortion of reality, and delusions.

F. The delusions can be
1. Jealous
    The jealousy is usually more persistent and profound than normal jealousy. There is usually some grain of truth in the pathological jealousy, but the constructs on which it rests are based on inadequate evidence. Shakespeare's Othello becomes furiously jealous of his innocent wife and his loyal lieutenant, and executes her with his own hands. When he learns of her innocence, he judges and executes himself.
2. Erotic
    These delusions may concern infidelity, sexual exploitation, change of sex, or the grandiose idea of being loved by someone

else (often a famous person who must keep the relationship secret).
  3. Grandiose

These are exalted delusions of having great power, influence, wealth, or of being a famous person. They seem to represent a regression to an earlier phase of development in which children regard themselves as omnipotent. An example is Cervantes' Don Quixote, whose windmill tilting was really combat against the villainous foe.
  4. Persecutory

In these delusions, paranoid persons feel watched, followed, slandered, or vilified, or believe their minds are being controlled or influenced by others or that they are being plotted against. An example is Herman Wouk's Captain Queeg, in *The Caine Mutiny*.
  5. Litigious

These delusions produce disputatiousness, contentiousness, fondness for litigation, or proneness to engage in lawsuits.
  G. Aside from the delusional system, there are no signs of mental disorder in the paranoid person. There is no withdrawal or regression (as in the schizophrenic disorders), nor any affective changes (as in affective disorders).

III. Prevalence

  A. Paranoid disorders are apparently rare. The *Diagnostic and Statistical Manual of Mental Disorders*, 3d ed. (*DSM*-III), states that one study of a large number of psychiatric hospital admissions showed that 0.4 percent or less were for paranoid disorders.
  B. Other studies have indicated that they may account for as much as 10 percent of hospital admissions.
  C. Recent studies indicate that such disorders are twice as common among women as among men.
  D. The proportion of unmarried and divorced people in this group is higher than in the general population.
  E. Paranoid disorders are more common among immigrant, minority, and migratory people.
  F. The paranoid is often of superior intellect.
  G. Paranoid disorders are said to be more common among the hard of hearing.

IV. Psychopathological factors

  A. The main causes are believed to be psychological (experiential).
  B. There is overuse of denial and projection as defenses against underlying conflicts, feelings of insecurity, repudiated impulses, and other conflictual factors.
  C. In the grandiose type, there is also overuse of rationalization.

D. As a child, the paranoiac was very likely suspicious, seclusive, secretive, and unable to develop any basic trust in others. (Often there was some basis for such feelings.)

E. As an adult, the paranoid is sensitive, distrustful, biased, unduly egocentric (narcissistic) and unyieldingly rigid.

F. In those with grandiose ideation, the behavior may be a response to a need to improve self-esteem or enhance prestige.

G. In general, the prepsychotic personality would be characterized as a paranoid (hypersensitive, rigid, suspicious, jealous, envious, excessively self-important, and tending to blame others and to ascribe evil motives to them).

H. Psychodynamically, there is projection of certain unacceptable impulses.
   1. According to Freud, these were repressed homosexual drives.
   2. According to Adler, these were repressed inferiority feelings.
   3. It is now thought that the unacceptable impulses may be any type of conflict, especially hostile and aggressive feelings.

V. Paranoia

A. Definition
   1. A psychotic disorder characterized by an elaborate, well-systematized, complex, intricate, logical, and well-fixed single delusional system and relatively good preservation of the remainder of the personality.
   2. Former synonyms were *true paranoia; paranoia vera.*

B. Historical note
   1. Literally, the term *paranoia* means thinking *beside* oneself.
   2. In antiquity, paranoia was synonymous with insanity.
   3. In the eighteenth century, the term was used to describe delusional and delirious conditions.
   4. In 1863, Kahlbaum limited the term to disorders with delusions of grandeur or persecution.
   5. The definition of paranoia vera was derived from Kraepelin's classification.
   6. The present definition is a chronic and stable delusional system of at least six months duration.

C. Prevalence
   1. This is a rare psychosis although there may be some unrecognized cases because the delusional system is well disguised.
   2. It is infrequent in youth because it is an insidiously developing condition which does not make itself obvious until later on.
   3. It is most commonly diagnosed between the ages of twenty-five and forty.

D. Psychopathology
   1. In the classical psychoanalytic formulation, paranoia represents a regression to an early anal phase.

2. Because paranoiacs are often of superior intellect, projection and rationalization are readily accessible to them.
3. For further details, see Psychopathological factors, the previous section of this chapter.
E. Symptomatology
   1. The other symptoms are related to the patient's delusional system.
   2. Clinical variants
      a. *Erotomania* is pathological preoccupation with erotic fantasies or activities. Most frequently found in women who fantasize a love relationship with a famous man.
      b. *Paranoid jealousy* is pathological jealousy. May follow an engagement, a marriage, or a narcissistic injury.
      c. *Megalomania* is a pathological preoccupation with delusions of omnipotence or wealth. Megalomaniacs may be convinced that they have unusual talents, without any confirming evidence.
   3. The delusion is usually not bizarre or even impossible.
   4. The degree to which the individuals may act on their delusion varies. They may only complain; they may become litigious; or they may become assaultive or homicidal.
F. Course and prognosis
   1. This is a chronic illness. The delusional system lasts at least six months.
   2. Nevertheless, progression may be halted at any stage of development.
   3. Since there is relatively good preservation of the personality aside from the elaborate, well-systematized, single delusional system, the patient's behavior is generally tolerated by society. Thus, most patients are never hospitalized but are regarded by others as "cranks" or eccentrics.
   4. Sometimes age diminishes the ability to follow through on the delusional system; such people may become less of a nuisance.
G. Treatment
   1. Most of the milder paranoiacs can make a marginal adjustment outside of the hospital. Thus, it is best to try to attempt treatment while the patient remains in the community.
   2. The therapist who can accept the paranoiac, at the same time clearly indicating non-agreement with the delusional system, may be of value in a supportive way to the patient. The therapist who is not skilled in dealing with such an individual may become a part of the patient's delusional system.
   3. Various neuroleptic drugs, especially the phenothiazines, butyrophenone or thioxinthene, may be of some help in modifying patients' delusional preoccupations or in assisting them to adapt more comfortably.

4. Sometimes the management of such cases is determined more by the needs of society than by the needs of the individual patient.
5. Few patients eventually require institutionalization.

VI. Acute paranoid disorder
A. This classification is for a paranoid condition of less than six months duration.

VII. Atypical paranoid disorder (paranoid state)
A. Definition
   1. An ill-defined group of reactions characterized by paranoid delusions that lack the logical systematization seen in paranoia but do not involve the regression, bizarreness, and deterioration found in paranoid schizophrenia. This is a residual category for paranoid disorders which are not classifiable elsewhere.
   2. Synonyms are *paraphrenia; paranoid condition; paranoid state; other paranoid disorders.*
   3. In the early nineteenth century, the clinical syndrome then known as *folly* (schizophrenia) was called paraphrenia.
B. Psychopathology
   See Psychopathological factors, earlier in this chapter.
C. Prevalence
   Most commonly seen in individuals who have recently changed their living or work situation, such as immigrants, refugees, prisoners of war, inductees into the military service, or young people leaving home for the first time. (*DSM*-III)
D. Symptomatology
   1. The onset is relatively abrupt.
   2. Delusions are not as well systematized as in paranoia, and are often modifiable and shifting.
   3. The patient does not act on the delusions in the persistent, militant fashion of the paranoiac.
   4. There is no evidence of personality deterioration, as there is in paranoid schizophrenia.
E. Prognosis
   1. The prognosis for these disorders is much more favorable than in paranoia, although these, too, may become recurrent.
   2. Occasionally, some great stress will occasion an acute paranoid episode that subsides when the stress is removed.
   3. The disorder rarely becomes chronic.
F. Treatment
   1. Psychotherapy is often helpful. The delusional symptoms are often responsive to therapeutic intervention.
   2. The paranoid person is usually distrustful and suspicious, and feels unloved. Thus, the therapist should be considerate and as

open and truthful as possible. The therapist should adopt an attitude of "I understand how you feel, but I don't agree with you, even though I like you."

3. Neuroleptic drugs, such as the phenothiazines, butyrophenones, thioxinthenes, often influence the delusional mentation favorably.

4. Electric convulsive therapy is occasionally helpful in shortening the duration of paranoid episodes.

G. Case example

Mr. H., a forty-year-old business executive, was admitted to the hospital mildly intoxicated and complaining that FBI agents were watching him because they suspected him of subversive activity.

He had first developed ideas of reference ten years before, while employed as an investigator for a governmental agency. Since that time, on several occasions, he had ideas that he was under surveillance by various investigating agencies.

VIII. Shared paranoid disorder
A. Definition
1. Shared paranoid disorder is a psychotic disorder in which two closely related people, usually members of the same family and who live in close and intimate association, share identical delusions.
2. A synonym is *folie à deux, induced,* or *communicated psychosis.* It has sometimes been called double insanity or psychosis of association.
3. Gralnick, who reviewed the English literature and reported on 103 cases in 1942, defined it as a "psychiatric entity characterized by the transference of delusional ideas or abnormal behavior from one person to one or more others who have been in close association with the primarily affected patient."
4. This is a rare condition, first described in 1877 by Laseque and Falret.

B. Psychopathology
1. A. A. Brill described the essential psychological process as unconscious identification.
   a. There is a communication of delusional ideas from one person to another (both of whom have been closely associated for a long period of time).
   b. It frequently involves a parent and child, husband and wife, or two sisters.
   c. The identification is a mutual phenomenon.
   d. Nothing is ever accepted by the secondary partner that is ego-alien. That is, the delusional material from the primary partner must resemble the unconscious fantasies and fit the defense mechanisms of the secondary partner.

e. The identification in *folie à deux* may be more akin to identification with the aggressor. As this was described by Anna Freud, identification with the aggressor is a defensive maneuver that protects the ego against real or feared aggression by allowing the individual to share in the power of the feared one.

2. The interdependence of the two partners is extreme; the identification is carried out in order to avoid a separation, which would be unendurable.
3. Heredity may be a predisposing factor.
4. Both persons usually have a long history of poor adjustment.
5. There is a close physical association between the two, who have usually lived in relative isolation and often in poverty.
6. The dominant partner is usually brighter.
7. In the prepsychotic relationship, the dominant partner is strongly dependent on the secondary partner and has few outside sources of gratification.
8. The dominant (primary) partner in the relationship is usually the one who has the primary psychotic disorder. The recipient (the secondary partner) of the induced delusions is often submissive, seclusive, and suspicious (i.e., schizoid), but develops these symptoms secondarily.
9. Since the disorder is usually characterized by delusions, the mechanism of projection is also operating. Because the primary partner is afraid of giving up the relationship, emerging hostility toward the secondary partner cannot be expressed directly. The defense used is the projection of the hostility onto an outsider in the form of paranoid delusions. The result is a paranoid psychosis.

C. Treatment
1. Separation of the two involved individuals.
2. Psychiatric treatment directed at the dominant person (primary partner), who has the primary psychotic symptoms. Treatment modalities should be those recommended for the patient's particular paranoid condition, and may include psychotherapy, neuroleptics, hospitalization, and maybe even electroconvulsive therapy.
3. The disorder of the recipient (secondary partner) may clear up without formal treatment, following separation from the primary psychotic partner.

D. Case example

A. T., a sixty-one-year-old single man, and V. T., his fifty-seven-year-old single sister with whom he had lived for many years, were referred to the court's psychiatric consultant for evaluation after they had both been found guilty of violation of the city fire ordinance on a number of occasions. Their offense consisted in hoarding a number of combustible items and trash in their home and on their premises. Neighbors complained, and the fire-prevention bureau, after repeatedly warning them about the combustible nature of the rubbish and other materials, filed a complaint.

The man, upon examination, showed flattened affect and was silly and inappropriate. He showed signs of schizoid behavior, including introversion, lack of verbal spontaneity and blocking, and was overly sensitive and suspicious. The schzoid and paranoid elements in his personality also became evident in the presentence study, where it was learned that he tended to place much of the blame for the collection of rubbish on his sister. His Minnesota Multiphasic Personality Inventory profile was clearly psychotic, showing elevations of the scales on the right-hand side.

The sister, at the time of the examination, seemed very frightened and kept asking if her brother could be present during the interview so he could "support me." She seemed preoccupied with her fantasy, but denied that she had hallucinations or delusions. She was evasive and defensive and had a number of "reasons" for hoarding trash in their home. From her description, she and her brother would collect a number of items and then spend much time going over them to try sorting out things that might have some value. Whenever she was questioned in detail about what valuable items might be in the trash or why the trash continued to accumulate, she would say, "You are trying to upset me."

Our conclusion was that the brother was the one primarily ill, that he had a paranoid, schizophrenic reaction, and that his sister had the same psychotic illness but, because she was the passive, submissive, suggestible one, she had developed it secondarily, through induction.

References

American Psychiatric Association. *Diagnostic and Statistical Manual of Mental Disorders.* 3d ed. Washington, D. C., 1978–1979.

Brill, A. A. *Fundamental Conceptions of Psychoanalysis.* New York: Arno Press, Inc., 1921.

Eaton, M. T., Jr.; Peterson, M. H.; and Davis, J. A. *Psychiatry.* 3d ed. Flushing, N.Y.: Medical Examination Publishing Company, 1976, chap. 15.

Freedman, A. M.; Kaplan, H. I.; and Sadock, B. J. *Modern Synopsis of Comprehensive Textbook of Psychiatry, Vol. 2.* Baltimore: Williams & Wilkins Company, 1976, chaps. 15, 26.

Gralnick, A. "Folie à Deux: The Psychosis of Association." *Psychiatric Quarterly.* 16 (1942):230.

Kolb, L. C. *Modern Clinical Psychiatry.* 9th ed. Philadelphia: W. B. Saunders Company, 1977, chap. 21.

Nicholi, A. M. *The Harvard Guide to Modern Psychiatry.* Cambridge: Harvard University Press, 1978, chap. 12.

Pulver, S. E., and Brunt, M. Y. "Deflection of Hostility and Folie à Deux." *Archives of General Psychiatry.* 5(1961):257–265.

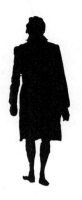

Alas, how right the ancient saying is:
We, who are old, are nothing else
but noise
And shape.
Like mimicries of dreams we go,
And have no wits although we think
us wise.

Euripides: *Aeolus (c. 423* B. C.**)**

Organic Mental Disorders

I. Definition
According to the *Diagnostic and Statistical Manual of Mental Disorders,* Third Edition (*DSM*-III), organic mental disorders are divided into two sections:
  A. Organic Mental Disorders
  Psychological or behavioral abnormality, associated with transient or permanent brain dysfunction, attributed to specific organic mental disorder (taken from the Mental Disorders section of *ICD*-9-CM), which can be etiologically related to the disorder by history, by physical examination as by laboratory tests (such as x-rays, brain scan, electroencephologram, and spinal fluid examination). Such mental disorders are:
    1. Senile and presenile dementias (primary degenerative dementia, or multi-infarct dementia)
    2. Substance induced disorder (such as alcohol, amphetamines, sedatives)
  B. Organic brain syndromes
  Psychological or behavioral abnormality associated with transient or permanent brain dysfunction, whose etiology or pathophysiological process is either noted as an additional diagnosis from outside the mental disorder section of *ICD*-9-CM or is unknown. Examples of such disorders are porphyria, certain endocrine dysfunctions, certain nutritional and deficiency states.
  C. An organic mental disorder is really an organic brain syndrome due to another organic mental disorder, whereas the term *organic brain syndrome* is reserved for the same symptomatology associated with other types of disorders.

II. Characteristics
  A. The fundamental process is the (presumed) destruction or damage of neurons (nerve cells).
  B. It is this damage, rather than the quality of the destructive process, that is responsible for the typical clinical picture.
  C. Strictly speaking, damage to the brain does not fully account for the occurrence of the abnormal behavior. Psychological and sociocultural factors also play a role.
    1. Psychological factors
    These include: (a) previous personality; (b) the manner in which the person previously coped with environmental stresses and internal conflicts; and (c) the manner of dealing with the organic deficit, which is determined by the person's adjustive patterns and coping mechanisms.
    2. Sociocultural factors
    These include: (a) the demands of the environment; (b) the psychosocial setting in which the illness develops; (c) the person's cultural background; and (d) the presence or absence of support from family and others.

D. Thus, senile changes in the brain (primary degenerative dementia) may produce confused and deteriorated behavior in one person, depressive symptoms in a second, paranoid behavior in a third, and have no appreciable affect on yet a fourth.

E. The reactions in organic mental disorders might be regarded as being released by the brain damage and superimposed upon it.

III. Prevalence

A. Organic mental disorders are common and may occur at any age.
   1. Some, such as senile dementia (primary degenerative dementia, senile onset), are found in late life.
   2. Others, such as Pick's disease (a presenile focal degenerative disease of the brain affecting the cerebral cortex, particularly the frontal lobes) or Alzheimer's disease (a presenile diffuse degenerative organic brain disease) are found in late middle life (primary degenerative dementia, presenile onset; or, multi-infarct dementia).
   3. Others, resulting from head injuries, are more commonly found in early life.
   4. Organic brain syndromes associated with infectious diseases, substance abuse, or alcohol abuse, may occur at almost any age.

B. Variable incidence
   1. Some organic mental disorders seem to be increasing in frequency, as, for example, senile dementia and normotensive hydrocephalus (a non-absorptive communicating type of hydrocephalus that develops in the absence of a demonstrable lesion). These are increasing because of the aging of the population.
   2. Others are decreasing in frequency as, for example, the organic brain syndrome associated with syphilis of the central nervous system (general paresis).

IV. Etiology

A. Any condition that causes cerebral tissue impairment may lead to organic mental disorder.

B. The potential causes of organic mental disorders are[1]
   1. Endocrine dysfunction
      a. Thyroid disease
      b. Parathyroid disease
      c. Adrenal dysfunction
      d. Hypoglycemia
   2. Metabolic and electrolytic abnormalities
      a. Liver disease
      b. Kidney disease

---

1. From G. C. Peterson, "Organic Brain Syndrome." Psychiatric Clinics of North America, Volume 1, No. 1, April, 1978.

   c. Lung disease

   d. SIADA acidosis, alkalosis

   e. Wilson's disease

   f. Porphyria

3. Nutritional and deficiency states
   a. Vitamin deficiencies such as thiamin, niacin, and vitamin B-12
   b. Iron deficiency
   c. Pernicious anemia

4. Drugs and medications
   a. Alcohol
   b. Various sedatives
   c. Anticholinergic drugs
   d. Steroids
   e. Amphetamines
   f. Anti-hypertensive drugs

5. Toxic conditions
   a. Heavy metal such as lead, mercury, arsenic, thalium
   b. Solvents
   c. Organophosphates

6. Infections
   a. Brain abcess
   b. CNS syphilis
   c. Meningoencephalitis
   d. Pneumonia
   e. Septicema

7. Post traumatic reactions
   a. Subural hematoma
   b. Normotensive hydrocephalis
   c. Contusion

8. Degenerative and "slow viral" diseases
   a. Alzheimer's disease
   b. Pick's disease
   c. Amyotropic lateral sclerosis
   d. Huntington's disease

9. Vascular disorders
   a. Hypertension
   b. Cerebral embolism and thrombosis
   c. Cerebral atherosclerosis
   d. Congestive heart failure

10. Neoplastic disorders
    a. Primary brain tumor
    b. Metastic cancer

11. Other causes
    a. Intractible seizures
    b. Status petit mal
    c. Remote effects of carcinoma
C. The most common organic brain disorders seen in clinical practice are the dementias, occurring in the geriatric population.

V. Symptomatology

A. There is usually some evidence of an organic factor from the history, physical, neurological, or laboratory examinations. For example, cerebral concussion or contusion in patients with skull fractures; paralysis, paresis, reflex or sensory changes in patients with brain tumors; urinary or blood chemistry changes in people who have had heavy metal poisoning; spinal fluid changes in patients with deliria caused by infectious illnesses; evidence of cerebral atrophy on computerized cranial tomography (CT scan) in patients with degenerative diseases such as Alzheimer's, Pick's, or senile dementia; history of excessive alcoholic intake in somebody with dementia associated with chronic alcoholism; history of exposure to some industrial toxic in toxic delirium.

B. The symptomatology associated with the various organic brain syndromes (modified from *DSM*-III).
   1. Delirium (acute brain syndrome)
      All the symptoms listed below develop over a short period of time, fluctuate rapidly, and are evidenced by physical, neurological, or laboratory examinations, or by a history of specific organic factors.
      a. Disturbance of attention, clouding of consciousness
      b. Disordered memory and orientation
      c. Sleep disturbance (reduced wakefulness or insomnia); or, drowsiness
      d. Perceptual disturbances (misinterpretations, illusions, or hallucinations)
      e. Increased or decreased psychomotor activity
      f. Incoherent speech
   2. Dementia (may be reversible, e.g., normotensive hydrocephalus)
      a. Memory impairment
      b. Deterioration of intellectual abilities
      c. Impairment of abstract thinking
      d. Impairment of judgment or impulse control
      e. Personality change
      f. Consciousness is not clouded
      g. Evidence of organic factor
   3. Amnestic syndrome
      a. Short-term but not immediate memory disturbance, in the absence of dementia or delirium

      b. A specific organic factor that is judged to be causally related to the disturbance

  4. Organic delusional syndrome (delusions predominate)
      a. Delusions in a full state of wakefulness and alertness
      b. Evidence from either physical examination, laboratory tests, or a history of a specific organic factor

  5. Organic hallucinosis (hallucinations predominate)
      a. Persistent or recurrent hallucinations in a state of full wakefulness and alertness
      b. Attributability to some clearly defined organic factor

  6. Organic affective syndrome
      a. Disturbance in mood closely resembling that seen in a depressive or manic episode
      b. Attributability to some clearly defined organic factor

  7. Organic personality syndrome
      a. Marked personality change (changes include emotional lability, impairment in impulse control; marked apathy and indifference; or suspiciousness or non-delusional paranoid sensitivity)
      b. Attributability to some organic factor

  8. Intoxication
      a. Recent ingestion and presence in the body of a toxic substance
      b. Maladaptive behavior during the waking state due to the effect of the substance on the central nervous system

  9. Withdrawal
    A substance-specific syndrome that follows cessation or reduction of intake of a substance that was previously regularly used by the individual to induce a state of intoxication

  10. Atypical or mixed organic brain syndrome
     Residual category reserved for syndromes that do not meet the criteria for any of the other organic brain syndromes, and in which there are maladaptive changes during the waking state

VI. Treatment

A. Treatment depends upon the underlying etiology. Treatment is directed at the underlying mental, medical or neurological disorder.

B. Certain medications are prescribed. For example, phenothiazines are prescribed for agitation accompanying senile behavior; benzodiazepines, during the withdrawal period from various substance use disorders; vasodilators, for patients who have vascular disorders of the brain. In many of these cases, only the smallest dose should be used, since patients with brain syndromes are frequently quite sensitive to these drugs.

C. Management of the patient's behavior frequently involves repeating simple explanations and giving help with orientation, as well as frequently adopting a reassuring attitude.

D. Patients who have deliria do better with constant light. Shadows and darkness increase their illusions and frighten them.

E. Some patients need protection from harming themselves or others.

VII. Case examples

A. Case example, withdrawal

A thirty-five-year-old man was admitted to the hospital for a leg injury. He gave a history of alcoholism dating back to age eighteen and said that he had been drinking at least one pint of whiskey daily for several months prior to admission.

The morning following admission, the nurses noted that he seemed confused and could not give the correct date or the name of the hospital. By late afternoon he appeared anxious and swept his hand along his torso and extremities as if brushing something off. On inquiry, he admitted to "seeing" tiny green animals crawling over his body. By late evening he was very excited and fearful, especially if left by himself in the darkened room. He was transferred to the psychiatric ward, where he recovered from the acute psychotic episode after two days.

In this case, note the history of substance use disorder (chronic alcoholism), the sudden onset of disorientation, mood change, and the vivid, visual hallucinations. Note also the rapid recovery from the acute episode.

B. Case example, delirium

A seventy-four-year-old man developed symptoms of enlarged prostate, or benign prostatic hyperthrophy (frequent urination, nocturia, dysuria, and urinary retention). The urinary retention became so severe that he had to be hospitalized.

Two days after admission, he became confused, disoriented, and unruly. He had visual hallucinations (e.g., he saw his son outside his hospital room) and was delusional (he was paranoid about some of the nurses and at times thought he was God). Examination revealed a markedly enlarged prostate gland and an elevated blood urea nitrogen (indicative of uremia). Following surgical resection of the enlarged prostate, his uremia cleared up and his mental symptoms disappeared.

Note that his symptoms were produced by uremia and disappeared when this was cleared up by treating the underlying cause of the uremia.

C. Case example, primary degenerative dementia, presenile onset

A forty-eight-year-old woman was brought to the hospital by her son, who said she was disoriented, showed poor judgment, was difficult to manage, and behaved in a childish manner. The onset of symptoms was noted two years earlier, when she first complained of impaired memory for recent events and forgot some of the routine tasks associated with her job as a receptionist. Very shortly after, she showed poor judgment in dealing with people and made obscene remarks to her colleagues. Because of this behavior, she was fired. At home, she progressively deteriorated: she became slovenly in dress, careless of excreta, and markedly disoriented. At the time of admission, she was incapable of carrying out even simple household tasks.

Examination revealed her to be completely disoriented about time and place. Recent and remote memory were totally defective. She was apathetic, disinterested, and passively cooperative. At times she seemed to be responding to auditory hallucinations. Physical and neurological examinations were essentially negative. A pneumoencephalogram (X-ray examination of the skull after replacing the cerebrospinal fluid with air) revealed findings compatible with generalized cerebral atrophy. She was transferred to a state hospital where her behavior progressively deteriorated.

Note the typical organic symptoms and their progressive nature, a result of the permanent and progressive cerebral atrophy. This generalized cerebral atrophy, occurring in middle life, is called Alzheimer's disease. The pathological changes in the brain are similar to those found in senile dementia.

D. Case example, primary degenerative dementia, senile onset

A seventy-six-year-old widow was admitted to the hospital complaining of memory loss and hallucinations. She had been well until about a year earlier, when her family first noticed that she was forgetful and had trouble remembering the date. Shortly, she began complaining about strange noises in her apartment. The family was not especially concerned by this complaint since they knew that one of her neighbors had frequent parties and that another kept a dog and other pets in his apartment. About four months before admission, the patient began complaining that her next-door neighbor was a gangster and accused him of shooting someone in his apartment. One week before admission, she went to the manager of the apartment building and complained about the people who were walking through her closed doors and windows. Her family was summoned and they brought her to the hospital.

Examination revealed her to be grossly disoriented about time and place. Both recent and remote memory were impaired. She had visual hallucinations (e.g., she saw dogs in her room) and was mildly suspicious of the staff. Physical and neurological studies were negative except for X-ray evidence of mild rheumatoid arthritis. After a few weeks, her hallucinations and delusions cleared up and she recognized that she had experienced a psychotic episode. At the time of her discharge two months later, she was still disoriented about time and had a fair amount of recent memory impairment. However, she was able to return to her apartment and adjust with only minimal supervision.

This is primary degenerative dementia, senile onset. Note the onset in late life of behavioral changes in the absence of any specific positive physical, neurological, or laboratory findings. The "improvement" following hospitalization is not unusual in this type of reaction although, as in this case, there is usually some residual permanent brain damage (disorientation and memory loss persisted after discharge).

References

American Psychiatric Association. *Diagnostic and Statistical Manual of Mental Disorders.* 3d ed. Washington, D. C., 1978–1979.

Freedman, A. M.; Kaplan, H. I.; and Sadock, B. J. *Modern Synopsis of Comprehensive Textbook of Psychiatry.* Vol. 2. Baltimore: Williams & Wilkins Company, 1976, chap. 18.

Goodwin, D. W., and Guze, S. B. *Psychiatric Diagnosis.* 2d ed. New York: Oxford University Press, 1979, chap. 10.

Kolb, L. C. *Modern Clinical Psychiatry.* 9th ed. Philadelphia: W. B. Saunders Company, 1977, chaps. 9–18.

Peterson, G. C. Organic Brain Syndrome in Symposium on Brain Disorders, *Psychiatric Clinics of North America* 1:21.

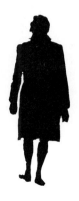

False facts are highly injurious to the progress of science, for they often endure long; but false views, if supported by some evidence, do little harm, for everyone takes salutory pleasure in proving their falseness.

Charles Robert Darwin: *Descent of Man (1871)*

Assessment of the Psychiatric Patient

By Shirley H. Mink, Ph.D., and Walter D. Mink, Ph.D.

I. Purposes of assessment

Assessment procedures play an important role in establishing a working diagnosis and planning a treatment program for a psychiatric patient. Systematic assessment contributes to establishing the probable etiology and course of the patient's disorder, designing the form of intervention, predicting and monitoring response to treatment, evaluating results of treatment, and following up the patient when intervention is terminated.

II. Areas of investigation

Assessment procedures elicit information about the following areas of the patient's condition and experience.

A. Current psychological functioning and symptom formation

B. Current life situation and sources of stress

C. Personal history, including critical developmental incidents

D. Personality structure and defenses (psychodynamics)

III. Methods of assessment

A. The interview

1. The interview is the most widely used assessment technique in psychiatric practice.

2. The interview provides not only factual information about the patient, but also an opportunity to observe such personal characteristics as appearance, manner, speech, and mode of interpersonal response.

3. Interviews with informants other than the patient provide independent information that may corroborate the patient's report or indicate important omissions and inconsistencies. This source of information is particularly important when patients may be without insight, delusional, confused, or otherwise inaccessible or uncooperative.

4. In psychiatric interviewing, the following points of inquiry are usually included.

   a. The presenting complaint

   b. History of present illness

   c. Nature of previous adjustment

   d. Educational, social, and occupational history

   e. Family and marital history

   f. Past medical history

B. Mental-status examination

The mental-status examination is a special form of assessment often conducted in conjunction with the history-taking interview. (Refer to section on symptom formation in mental disorders.) It provides the following kind of outline for recording the interviewer's descriptions of the patient's behavior.

1. Mental content

   a. This consists of the thoughts, concerns, and trends that are uppermost in the patient's mind.

b. Disturbances of content include delusions, hallucinations, obsessions, and phobias.

2. Sensorium and intellect
   a. The degree of the patient's awareness and the level of his or her functioning.
   b. Disturbances of orientation, memory, retention, attention, information, and judgment can be elicited with standardized questions and test materials.

3. Stream of thought
   a. This includes the quantitative and qualitative aspects of the patient's verbal communication.
   b. Disturbances include over and underproductivity, disconnectedness, unintelligibility, and incoherence.

4. Emotional tone
   a. This includes the patient's report of subjective feelings (mood or affect) and the examiner's observations of facial expression, posture, and attitude.
   b. Disturbances include both quantitative deviations (elation, depression, apathy) and incongruence (disagreement among the patient's subjective report, behavior, and mental content).

5. Attitude, manner, and behavior
   a. Appearance, dress, facial expression, activity, posture, and demeanor are noted.
   b. Disturbances include deviations of degree of activity, mannerisms, distortions of motility, and uncooperativeness.

6. Insight
   This means the degree to which the patient can appreciate the nature of his or her condition and the need for treatment.

7. Instruments
   Instruments have been developed to standardize the mental-status examination.
   a. The Mental Status Schedule is an example of such an instrument. A trained interviewer, guided by a standard interview schedule, administers the tests and scores the responses at intervals during the session.
   b. The Inpatient Multidimensional Psychiatric Scale provides a systematic way for rating the behavior of severely disturbed psychiatric patients.

C. Physical and neurological examination
   A routine physical and neurological examination is an essential part of general psychiatric assessment. Special diagnostic and laboratory procedures are used when organic impairment is suspected.

IV. Psychological testing

The development of psychological measurements of human characteristics has provided many tools for psychiatric assessment.

A. Variability from person to person is a commonly acknowledged aspect of many characteristics of human behavior. Psychological testing is based on the assumption that this variability can be measured.

B. Technically, a test is a systematic way to compare the behavior of two or more persons.

C. The development, administration, and interpretation of the tests most widely used in psychiatric assessment require special skill and training. The American Psychological Association has established ethical standards for the distribution and use of psychological tests.

D. Criteria for evaluation of psychological tests

While psychological tests vary in content, purpose, and range of application, they are generally evaluated by the following criteria.

1. *Reliability,* the consistency with which a test measures what it proposes to measure.

2. *Validity,* the accuracy with which a test fulfills its purpose of prediction, selection, or classification.

3. *Standardization,* the establishment of responses of reference groups so that individual performance may be compared with the performance of an appropriate group.

E. Other characteristics of tests

1. Individual versus group

Some tests can be administered to only one person at a time (individual tests); others are administered to a number of persons at one time (group tests).

2. Standardization of administration

Tests vary in the degree to which the tester must follow a prescribed procedure.

3. Objectivity

Tests vary in the degree to which interpretation is required in the scoring of responses. An objective test is one whose scoring minimizes differences among different scorers.

4. Form of response

Some tests require a specific form of response (e.g., true-false); others permit open-end responses (e.g., sentence completion).

F. There are various kinds of psychological tests. In the ensuing sections, we shall describe the most important of the following types.

1. Intelligence tests

2. Personality tests

   a. Objective personality tests

   b. Projective techniques of measuring personality

3. Vocational tests
4. Neuropsychological tests
5. Behavioral assessment

V. Intelligence tests

A. The "intelligence" measured by intelligence tests is considered to be a general, relatively stable capacity to learn and deal effectively with one's environment.

B. Intelligence is assumed to be normally distributed in the population.

C. The results of intelligence tests are frequently reported in terms of an IQ (intelligence quotient) score.

   1. The IQ score indicates the position of a person's intelligence test performance relative to the average performance of his or her age group. The average IQ is 100.
   2. The commonly used classification of intelligence includes:
      a. Very superior, IQ 130 or more
      b. Superior, 120–129
      c. Bright-normal, 110–119
      d. Average, 90–109
      e. Dull-normal, 80–89
      f. Borderline, 70–79
      g. Mental defective, 69 or less.[1]

D. In psychiatric practice, the intelligence test is used to
   1. Aid in establishing the diagnosis of mental retardation
   2. Assess the effects of brain damage
   3. Assess effective intellectual performance in psychiatric disorders
   4. Define a patient's intellectual resources for educational and vocational adjustment

E. Since intelligence is, to a substantial degree, defined culturally, tests of intelligence reflect competencies and achievements that are considered important for success in the culture. Interpretations of test results should be made with full consideration of the appropriateness of the test for the particular person who is tested.

F. Major intelligence tests in current usage
   1. The New Revised Stanford-Binet (1960)
      a. Widely used, individually administered intelligence test for children and for the assessment of mental retardation.
      b. Serves as the standard for comparison with other tests of intellectual ability
      c. Composed of various tasks and problems organized by year levels arranged from two years to superior adult.
      d. The problems successfully solved at each year level are totalled and the sum is expressed as a Mental Age Score and has an IQ score equivalent.

---

1. The American Association of Mental Deficiency classifies four categories of mental retardation: mild, moderate, severe, and profound.

e. Test has proved useful in the prediction of school achievement.

f. Examples of types of tasks include vocabulary, memory span for digits, words, and sentences, reasoning, comprehension, copying geometric figures, etc. Verbal ability is strongly emphasized.

g. Test is of limited usefulness with adults because it was standardized primarily with children and is composed of tasks that are more appropriate for children.

h. The test choice for reliable assessment of the extreme ranges of intelligence, both low and high.

2. The Wechsler Adult Intelligence Scale (WAIS)

a. The most widely used individually administered intelligence test for adults and the standard against which other adult intelligence tests are compared.

b. Composed of a series of subtests organized into a verbal scale and a performance scale.

c. Verbal subtests are
   (1) Information
   (2) Comprehension
   (3) Similarities
   (4) Arithmetic
   (5) Digit span
   (6) Vocabulary

d. Performance subtests are
   (1) Picture arrangement
   (2) Picture completion
   (3) Block design
   (4) Object assembly
   (5) Digit symbol

e. The test yields three IQ scores:
   (1) Verbal scale IQ
   (2) Performance scale IQ
   (3) Full scale IQ.

f. Differences between verbal and performance IQ scores may sometimes be of diagnostic value. However, differences in the pattern of subtest scores have not proved to be of any consistent diagnostic significance.

g. There are two other forms of the Wechsler Intelligence Scale:
   (1) Wechsler-Bellevue Form I, which is now rarely used.
   (2) Wechsler-Bellevue Form II, which is the retest instrument for the WAIS.

h. Two forms of the test have also been developed for children.
   (1) The Wechsler Intelligence Scale for Children (WISC) is designed for children ages five to fifteen and is the most widely used intelligence test for children.
   (2) The Wechsler Pre-School and Primary Scale of Intelligence (WPPSI) has been developed for children ages four to six-and-one-half.
3. Special individually administered intelligence tests have been devised for use with illiterate, blind, deaf, and other handicapped persons who would not be accurately tested on the standard tests.
4. Group tests
   a. Large numbers of paper-and-pencil group tests of intelligence are available and are used primarily in schools and personnel departments in business and industry.
   b. While these tests generally yield IQ scores, it may be more meaningful to reserve the use of the term *IQ* for the individually administered intelligence test.

VI. Personality tests
A. There is a great variety of personality measures that differ in form, content, and interpretation.
B. Some personality measures are attempts to assess personality traits or characteristics, others are attempts to reveal a pattern of personality dynamics (e.g., motives, defenses, conflicts).
C. Personality measures can be divided roughly into objective tests and projective techniques.

VII. Objective personality tests
A. Objective tests usually take the form of questionnaires or rating scales; the subjects respond to the items according to how characteristic they are of their experience and behavior.
B. Tests are administered and scored in a standardized way; the results are expressed in numerical scores.
C. Since objective tests are a form of self-report, they are open to faking and dissimulation. However, their ease of administration permits the testing of large numbers of persons by staff other than special clinical personnel.
D. The Minnesota Multiphasic Personality Inventory (MMPI) is the most widely used objective personality test in psychiatric practice in the United States. It consists of 550 true-false items.
   1. Validity scales
      There are four special scales that are scored to indicate response tendencies and test-taking attitudes that might make interpretations of the test doubtful.

2. Clinical scales
   a. Responses are scored in terms of correspondence to the responses of diagnosed psychiatric groups. The clinical scales can be scored for hypochondriasis, depression, hysteria, psychopathic deviate, paranoia, psychasthenia, schizophrenia, and mania.
   b. Two other scales, masculinity-femininity and social introversion, are typically used in connection with the clinical scales.
3. Other scales
In addition to the clinical scales, many research scales have been developed for special purposes or to measure other personality characteristics (e.g., dependency, ego-strength).
4. Interpretation
Interpretation of the test is based on the pattern of scores. In recent years, standardized interpretations have been developed for common patterns. Computer programs can now be used to score the test and produce analyses of the profiles of the scores.
5. Evaluation
A sizable literature (more than three thousand articles and books) has been developed around the MMPI. Reviews of this literature indicate that the test is sufficiently reliable and valid for many applications.

VIII. Projective techniques of measuring personality
  A. Characteristics of projective measures
    1. The term *projective* implies that the patients "project" their personalities into the responses they make.
    2. The materials of most projective methods are unstructured or ambiguous; thus, they require that the patient organize them in some imaginative way.
    3. The patients have considerable freedom in their responses.
    4. It is assumed that the way the patients respond reveals emotional and motivational factors which are characteristic of them, though perhaps unconsciously.
    5. The interpretation of the responses is subjective and is usually based on the theoretical assumptions of the interpreter. This leads to less consistent interpretation than is obtained with objective tests.
    6. Both the administration and interpretation of projective tests require special training and experience.
  B. The Rorschach method
  The Rorschach is the best known and most widely used of the projective techniques.

1. Administration
   a. The materials consist of ten "inkblots." Patients are asked to describe what each one looks like. They may offer as many responses to each card as they wish.
   b. Following the administration of the test, the examiner questions the subject about the response made, asking him or her to indicate the location on the inkblot that prompted the response and to say what about the blot (e.g., shape, color, texture) contributed to the response.
2. Scoring
   Responses are scored according to:
   a. Content (e.g., human, animal, object, X-ray);
   b. The area of the blot included in the content (whole blot or a particular section of it); and
   c. The characteristics of the blot (e.g., color, shading, and shape) that determined the content.
3. Interpretation
   a. Interpretation is based on the assumed personal significance of the responses, as well as on characteristic ways in which the patients organize their responses.
   b. A theory about Rorschach responses relates such factors as the use of color and the interpretation of movement to forms of psychopathology.
   c. Interpretation rests heavily on psychoanalytic, especially Jungian, theory.
4. Evaluation
   A tremendous literature (more than three thousand articles and books) pertaining to the Rorschach has developed. Reviews of this literature consistently raise serious questions about the reliability and validity of this instrument.
C. Thematic Apperception Test (TAT)
   1. This test consists of twenty illustrations. The patient is asked to tell a story about the content of each picture.
   2. Stories are interpreted in terms of their themes, the handling of motivational states, the resolution of conflicts, the ways in which interpersonal relations are presented, and the extent to which patients identify themselves with the characters they describe.
   3. Several complete methods of scoring have been developed. They require special training.
D. Other projective techniques
   1. A large number of other techniques, involving word association, sentence completion, drawing, and storytelling have been devised.

2. They have in common the assumption that imaginative productions and fantasy yield important clues to personality.

IX. Vocational tests

A. Since the problems faced by some patients involve vocational maladjustment and dissatisfaction, vocational testing can contribute important information to a total treatment program. In general, vocational tests are of two types, measurements of aptitude and measures of interests.

B. Aptitude tests
  1. Available tests measure a variety of special aptitudes and abilities such as clerical ability, mechanical ability, spatial reasoning, hand-and-finger dexterity, and rate of manipulation.
  2. Norms permit comparison of individual scores with scores of representative occupational groups.

C. Interest tests
  1. Interest tests permit the comparison of the individual's interests with the interests of persons representative of a number of professions and occupations.
  2. The most commonly used vocational interest test for adults is the Strong-Campbell Interest Inventory (SCII).
  3. The correlation of the individual's interests with those of representative members of particular occupations has been shown to be strongly related to job satisfaction.

D. Professional and managerial tests
  1. The assessment of aptitude for professional and managerial occupations is more complex.
  2. It involves the assessment of a variety of factors, including information, intellect, personality, attitudes, and interests.
  3. These tests are not considered as valid as the simpler tests of aptitudes and interests.

X. Neuropsychological tests

A. The assessment of intellectual deficit and the differentiation of organic brain conditions is often a problem in psychiatric diagnosis.

B. More accurate assessments of deficits due to brain damage can be made if earlier test scores, with which present performance can be compared, are available. This is seldom possible.

C. There are some tests that compare performance that is more sensitive to brain damage (e.g., abstract reasoning), with performance that is less affected (e.g., vocabulary).

D. Other tests have been designed to assess specific aspects of brain function such as memory, perception, language use, and motor coordination.

E. Tests of brain damage sometimes yield helpful diagnostic hypotheses. However, their further usefulness depends on the success of research into the neurological and behavioral correlates of brain activity.

XI. Behavioral assessment

A. The increase in the application of behavioral concepts and methodology to clinical practice has been accompanied by the elaboration of techniques of assessing behavior.

B. In behavioral assessment, emphasis is placed on the objective description of behavior and on the environmental events and contexts that were antecedent and consequent to the behavior being investigated.

C. While some behavioral assessment is similar to traditional methods of investigation, the purpose is to elicit information about characteristic reactions to situations with a minimum of inference, rather than to elicit information about psychodynamic determinants.

D. The emphasis on objective descriptions of current behavior makes behavioral assessment useful to the eclectic practitioner.

E. Techniques of behavioral assessment include
 1. Interviewing
    a. The interview is used to obtain self-reported information about problem behavior and the circumstances that influence it.
    b. The interview also provides an opportunity to raise and test hypotheses about the events that may interfere with or support attempts to modify the patient's behavior.
 2. Inventories and scales
    a. Self-reported information can be obtained with questionnaires and "behavior-and-situation" check-lists.
    b. A variety of special-purpose devices has been developed, but as yet no standard procedures have emerged.
 3. Observation
    a. Both direct and indirect techniques have been used to obtain information about behavior.
    b. While indirect methods are preferred because they do not, in themselves, influence behavior, they may not be feasible in most clinical situations.
 4. Simulation
    a. This technique is also called role playing.
    b. "Real-life" situations are constructed, and patients are asked to assume a role.
    c. By observing how the role is played, the therapist is enabled to observe the patient's characteristic modes of response.

        d. Investigation of similarities in behavior in natural and simulated situations suggests that there is a fair degree of consistency.

    5. Assessment of therapeutic change

        a. All the methods described in this section contribute to the modification of problem behavior by directing the patient's attention to the frequency with which it occurs and the contexts in which it is most likely to occur.

        b. Self-observation and simulation provide the patient as well as the therapist with opportunities to modify and monitor changes in behavior.

        c. In behavior therapy, the problems are formulated in terms of behavior that is to be altered. Thus, techniques of behavioral assessment can be used to determine the frequency and consistency of behavioral change and, thus, provide an index of success of treatment.

XII. Trends in psychiatric assessment

A. Emphasis is shifting from the use of assessment to establish a specific diagnosis to its use in defining problems and developing a program of intervention.

B. Emphasis is also shifting from the assessment of psychopathology or deficiencies to an inclusion of areas of competency.

C. Insofar as much behavior seems to be influenced by special characteristics of the environment, more attention is being paid to the assessment of situations and the way the person responds to and influences them.

D. As patients play a more active role in their own treatment and management, self-assessment procedures assume importance.

E. Assessment is becoming an essential component of therapeutic intervention, from its initial stages through follow-up.

F. In the multiaxial classification proposed in the *Diagnostic and Statistical Manual of Mental Disorders,* 3d ed.(*DSM*-III), assessment is not only of symptoms (Axis I), personality (Axis II), and physical disorders (Axis III), but also of experiential and situational sources of stress (Axis IV) and competence or level of adaptive functioning (Axis V).

G. Programs and institutions are now being assessed, so that the progress of the individual patient is being viewed in relation to the effectiveness of programs in medical and social institutions.

References

American Psychiatric Association. *Diagnostic and Statistical Manual of Mental Disorders.* 3d ed. Washington, D. C., 1978–1979.

American Psychological Association. *Standards for Educational and Psychological Tests and Manuals.* Washington, D. C., 1974.

Buros, O. K., ed. *The Seventh Mental Measurements Yearbook.* Highland Park, N. J.: Gryphon Press, 1972.
————. *Intelligence Tests and Reviews.* Highland Park, N. J.: Gryphon Press, 1975.
Cone, J. D., and Hawkins, R. P., eds. *Behavioral Assessment.* New York: Brunner/Mazel, 1977.

Cronbach, L. *Essentials of Psychological Testing.* New York: Harper & Row, Publishers, 1960.
Dahlstron, W. G., Welsh, G. S., and Dahlstrom, L. E. *An MMPI Handbook. Clinical Interpretation,* vol. 1. Rev. ed. Minneapolis: University of Minnesota, 1972.
Rabin, A. I., ed. *Projective Techniques in Personality Assessment.* New York: Springer, 1968.

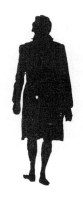

Canst thou not minister to a mind
   diseas'd;
Pluck from the memory a rooted
   sorrow;
Raze out the written troubles of the
   brain;
And, with some sweet oblivious
   antidote,
Cleanse the staff'd bosom of that
   perilous matter
Which weighs upon the heart?

Shakespeare: *Macbeth*, **Act V
(c.1606)**

Treatment in Psychiatry

I. Introduction

A. Although reference has been made to types of treatment throughout the chapters on the various clinical syndromes, an attempt is made here to list in one place the various therapies that are available in psychiatry.

B. In the past, much treatment has been empirical and has not been scientifically evaluated. This is especially true of the various psychotherapies, because much of what has been written about them has been based solely on opinion and clinical experience. In recent years, there have been reports about the effect of various pharmacological therapies on the affective and schizophrenic disorders; these have been controlled studies, using the double-blind technique.

C. Treatment in psychiatry can be grouped into eight broad divisions—
1. Individual psychotherapy
2. Group psychotherapy
3. Family therapy
4. Somatic therapy (electroconvulsive therapy and psychosurgery)
5. Pharmacotherapy (chemotherapy)
6. Management therapy
7. Behaviorial therapy
8. Humanistic therapy

II. Psychotherapy

A. Introduction
1. Definition
   a. In the broad sense, many things that are done to or for a patient may have a psychotherapeutic effect.
   b. As defined in the more traditional sense in *A Psychiatric Glossary,* psychotherapy is "a process in which a person who wishes to change symptoms or problems in living or is seeking personal growth, enters, implicitly or explicitly, into a contract to interact in a prescribed way with a psychotherapist."[1]
2. Types of individual psychotherapy
   Psychotherapy can be divided into
   a. Psychoanalysis
   b. Uncovering therapy (intensive psychotherapy, investigative therapy)
   c. Hypnotherapy
   d. Supportive psychotherapy
3. Psychiatrists more or less agree on the aims of psychotherapy, but are less generally agreed about what it is able to accomplish.

1. Definition from *A Psychiatric Glossary,* 5th ed., American Psychiatric Association, Washington, D.C., 1980.

4. What type of patient will benefit from psychotherapy is not always clear. Most patients with anxiety disorders and some of the somatoform disorders would probably be considered candidates for psychotherapy. If they did not respond, some other therapy, such as chemotherapy, would probably be recommended. Probably many of the schizophrenias would be treated with neuroleptics and supportive therapy, and most of the affective disorders would be treated with combinations of chemotherapy and psychotherapy.
5. The therapist-patient relationship
   Of major importance in psychotherapy is the therapist-patient relationship. Whether or not psychotherapy is effective depends a great deal on the nature and quality of this relationship. Significant elements in this therapeutic relationship are
   a. Rapport
      (1) *A Psychiatric Glossary* defines *rapport* as "The feeling of harmonious accord and mutual responsiveness that contributes to the patient's confidence in the therapist and willingness to work cooperatively."[2]
      (2) Rapport is important in any treatment relationship, regardless of whether the patient is being treated for an emotional or a physical illness.
      (3) It is probably the single most effective therapeutic tool a physician has.
      (4) Some therapists speak of the "therapeutic alliance," which involves the primarily conscious and rational aspects of the treatment relationship. It is an agreement to work toward a mutual therapeutic goal.
      (5) Whatever treatment modality is used, *confidentiality* is an essential element of the relationship.
   b. Transference
      (1) Transference is the patient's unconscious attachment to the therapist (or others involved in the patient's treatment) of feelings and attitudes that were originally related to important figures (e.g., parents, siblings) in early life.
      (2) Transference can become so intense that it leads to the development of a "transference neurosis," a state in which early feelings and attitudes make up the bulk of the patient's feelings toward the physician.

2. Definition from *A Psychiatric Glossary,* 5th ed., American Psychiatric Association, Washington, D.C., 1980.

(3) *Countertransference* is the therapist's unconscious or conscious emotional reaction to the patient.

    (a) Feelings arising from the therapist's unresolved underlying conflicts may at times become intense and interfere with an understanding of the patient.

    (b) It is especially important that a therapist recognize any underlying negative countertransference.

    (c) Sometimes countertransference can be used diagnostically and therapeutically. For example, irritability or hostility in a therapist may be induced by fear in the patient; if the therapist is aware of the countertransference, he or she may more directly and correctly help the patient identify the underlying conflicts, recognize the fear, and resolve the issues behind it.

(4) Both positive and negative feelings are involved in transference and countertransference.

  c. Resistance

    (1) Resistance arises from the conscious or unconscious psychological forces in the patient that oppose bringing repressed (unconscious) material into consciousness.

    (2) Resistance is encountered in all forms of therapy, but is especially noted in individual psychotherapy.

    (3) It represents a mobilization of underlying defenses to resist treatment.

    (4) In any given situation, the physician must decide whether to leave the patient's resistance intact or to try to reduce it.

6. The choice of psychotherapeutic technique is determined to some extent by the type of disorder the patient has, but is often decided by the therapist's theoretical orientation (see the various concepts of personality development in the chapter, "Psychodynamic Concepts").

B. Psychoanalysis

  1. As noted in the chapter, "Psychodynamic Concepts," *psychoanalysis* means a theory of personality development, a method of research, and a system of treatment. It was originally developed by Sigmund Freud.

  2. As a treatment technique, it is defined in *A Psychiatric Glossary* as follows: "Through analysis of *free associations* and

interpretation of dreams, emotions and behavior are traced to the influence of *repressed instinctual drives* and *defenses against them in the unconscious.*"[3]

3. Because it involves a large expenditure of time, feeling, and money, psychoanalysis has only a limited place in the treatment of most mental disorders. However, the insights gained from it have been extremely helpful in the other forms of psychotherapy.

C. Uncovering therapy

1. *Uncovering therapy* is also called *intensive psychotherapy, insight psychotherapy,* and *investigative therapy.* Its purpose is to produce insight by uncovering conflicts, chiefly unconscious, so they can be dealt with more effectively.

2. Transference and countertransference are particularly important and must be dealt with.

3. Such treatment includes psychoanalytic therapy (which makes use of the insights of psychoanalysis) and psychobiological therapy (which makes use of the Meyerian, distributive analysis).

   a. Psychoanalytic therapy

   (1) As used by psychoanalysts, uncovering involves the exploration of the unconscious, chiefly through free association, which the *Psychiatric Glossary* defines as "the spontaneous uncensored verbalizations by the patient of whatever comes to mind."[4]

   (2) Dream material is often evaluated for clues to unconscious feelings, and interpretations are made to the patient.

   (3) Resistance (see above) must be recognized and dealt with.

   (4) Of major importance in this type of therapy is the therapist's ability to be a meaningful listener.

   (5) Interpretation is an integral part of this type of therapy. Interpretations may be made either of currently operating psychodynamic factors or of psychogenic forces. (The latter is focused on the relationship between current reactive states and past emotion.) Interpretation also helps to reduce resistance.

   (6) Correlation (reconstruction) is also employed to help relate past, repressed conflicts to current situations.

---

3. Definition from *A Psychiatric Glossary,* 5th ed., American Psychiatric Association, Washington, D.C., 1980.
4. Definition from *A Psychiatric Glossary,* 5th ed., American Psychiatric Association, Washington, D.C., 1980.

(7) "Working through" follows the development of insight and comprises a major portion of the treatment time. It includes repeated exploration of the insight gained through interpretation.

b. Psychobiological therapy

(1) Psychobiological therapy involves a critical examination and evaluation of *conscious* forces in the patient's personality development and emotional problems (i.e., the patient attempts to analyze and synthesize *consciously*).

(2) Elements of psychoanalytic therapy are also often used.

(3) As a matter of fact, most psychotherapists use an eclectic (the best from different systems) approach, combining psychoanalytic, psychobiological and various other approaches.

c. Case examples, uncovering therapy

(1) A forty-five-year-old widower complained of impotence. After three interviews, it became obvious that his symptom resulted from two important factors: (a) his guilt over having rejected his wife because she was physically unattractive; (b) the guilt was reactivated when he was sexually aroused.

His impotence was a protection against a second marriage to a woman he was dating but did not wish to marry. In this case, the conflicts were relatively superficial and readily accessible to the therapist. His symptom cleared up when he recognized the dynamic factors and broke off his relationship with the woman.

(2) A twenty-five-year-old man had consulted many physicians for palpitation, tachycardia, precordial pain, and apprehension. Each time, physical and laboratory examinations revealed no evidence of cardiac disease. Although he worried about his heart, his symptoms were typical of anxiety disorder.

During the first interview, it became apparent that his symptoms were related to his feelings about his father, but it was not until he had been seen for twelve sessions that he was able to see the relationship between his own symptoms and his father's heart attack a year earlier. When he did see that the onset of his own symptoms followed his father's heart attack and that his anxiety was being perpetuated by his guilt over his unconscious wish for his father's death, his symptoms disappeared.

(3) A thirty-year-old housewife had repeated episodes of parthesias, dizziness, and pains in her arms. These had begun shortly after her marriage and seriously

handicapped her. After about fifty hours of psychotherapy, she was able to recognize that these symptoms always developed when she felt rejected by her husband. This rejection awakened the underlying feelings that she had had when her father rejected her. When she recognized this, her symptoms cleared up.

The conflict here was unconscious and hence not as immediately available. Uncovering therapy brought the conflict to light.

D. Hypnotherapy

Some psychiatrists use hypnosis as a means of facilitating psychotherapy. It is often used to help people learn how to relax, and is occasionally employed to eliminate certain symptoms of psychogenic etiology (e.g., acute conversion symptoms).

E. Supportive psychotherapy

1. Supportive psychotherapy deals predominantly with conscious material and is centered chiefly on bolstering the individual's strength and assets. It reinforces healthy defenses and is based primarily on the therapist-patient relationship, including the so-called therapeutic alliance. Unlike uncovering psychotherapy, the focus tends to be on current problems; probing into the unconscious past is avoided.

2. The treatment objectives are usually limited. It is usually indicated for patients with acute emotional upheavals (e.g., anxiety disorders, depressive disorders) or for patients with acute psychotic decompensation.

3. Techniques include reassurance, unburdening, environmental modification, persuasion, and clarification.

a. Reassurance

Reassurance is the imparting or restoration of confidence and freeing the patient from fear and anxiety. It does not mean false reassurance. Reassurance cannot be imparted if the therapist is not herself or himself assured.

(1) Physical, laboratory, and X-ray examinations may relieve a person's anxiety about significant organic illness, and hence be reassuring.

(2) Examples of psychological reassurance include assuring panicky or obsessive-ruminative persons who fear serious mental breakdown that they will not lose their minds; assuring parents that the hostile and aggressive feelings they occasionally have about their children are not abnormal and will not lead to physical abuse; explaining to acutely depressed persons that their illness will be resolved.

b. Unburdening
  (1) *Unburdening* is the therapeutic release of feelings through conscious, free expression. This is "getting it off the chest." It is also called *ventilation* and *catharsis*.
  (2) It serves two purposes: (a) sharing, which helps "dilute" the feelings; and (b) self-punishment by revealing oneself.
  (3) For example, a sixty-year-old woman was finally able to tell the doctor how she had been emotionally clutching onto her thirty-five-year-old married daughter. After unburdening herself of this fact, which she had never before been able to verbalize, she was able to take the first major steps to release the hold on her daughter.

c. Environmental modification
  (1) *Environmental modification*, also called, *environmental manipulation*, means altering the environment so as to relieve the patient's symptoms and distress.
  (2) Caution must be exercised lest this type of treatment be misused.
  (3) Examples are providing a temporary homemaker or housekeeper for an anxious or depressed mother whose symptoms are aggravated by her responsibility for her young children; placing a patient in the relatively neutral environment of a hospital; placing a runaway child in a foster home until the parents can work out the marital conflicts that contributed to the running away; advising a vacation for a widower whose grief has been unduly prolonged.

d. Persuasion
  (1) *Persuasion* is direct suggestion, inducement, or entreatment in an effort to influence a patient's behavior.
  (2) Examples include asking a person who seems to be becoming psychologically dependent on alcohol for relaxation to try jogging, bicycling, or some other kind of physical exercise; asking a spouse to modify his or her behavior and attitudes if the patient for some reason is unable to do this (this example also includes the element of environmental modification).

e. Clarification
  (1) *Clarification* is a process by which the physician helps patients to understand their feelings and behavior and to gain a clearer picture of reality.

(2) Examples include pointing out to an agitated and depressed patient that a period of hospitalization will not worsen the condition; showing a paranoid patient how he or she is projecting; pointing out to a married person the rejecting behavior of a spouse who is really seeking a dissolution of the marriage.

III. Group psychotherapy

A. *Group psychotherapy* is defined in *A Psychiatric Glossary* as the "application of psychotherapeutic techniques to a group, including utilization of interactions of members of the group."[5]

B. Although it is sometimes used as the sole psychotherapeutic modality, it is most commonly used in conjunction with individual psychotherapy and other types of psychiatric treatment.

C. The groups are usually composed of one therapist and six or eight patients, who may be homogeneous in some way or heterogeneous. The sessions last about ninety minutes.

D. This type of psychotherapy has its origins in observations made by Sigmund Freud (in 1919) of the dynamics of the interplay between individuals in a group setting. There is a definite pattern of interaction between the various members of a group that facilitates the therapeutic process. The group provides an opportunity for developing personal insights as well as testing out new methods of coping and relating in a controlled type of environment.

E. The group process
Three stages characterize the life of the group, bringing specific issues into focus and dominating group interaction.
1. In the first phase, the patient is concerned about whether she or he will be accepted as a part of the group.
2. In the second phase, the patient is concerned with issues of autonomy, that is, becoming an independent person within the group.
3. In the third stage, the patient deals with the issues of sharing and equality.

F. There was a time when group psychotherapy was considered an expedient, a way to involve a greater number of patients, but this is no longer felt to be true.
1. For many patients, it is superior to individual psychotherapy.
2. The techniques used closely parallel those used in individual psychotherapy, and they vary with the aims of the therapist and the type of patient. That is, groups may be conducted by nonparticipating therapists (the psychoanalytic model), the

5. Definition from *A Psychiatric Glossary,* 5th ed., American Psychiatric Association, Washington, D.C., 1980.

very active therapists one sees in counselling, or any of the possible variants in between.

   G. There are several different types of groups.

      1. Since 1960, a number of variations of group therapy have emerged. They emphasize the usefulness of social processes in increasing self understanding, improving relationships, and developing human potentialities; such procedures can be useful adjuncts to psychiatric treatment.

      2. However, the variety of group procedures that is available may be confusing to many people; no "consumer's guide" is available and care must be exercised in evaluating the appropriateness of a group for oneself.

   H. Self-help groups

      1. *Self-help groups* are groups without professionally trained leaders, in which the group experience does not uncover basic conflicts but does offer new shared experiences to the patient.

      2. Alcoholics Anonymous (AA) and the substance abusers groups are effective self-help groups.

IV. Family therapy

   A. Description

      1. Family therapy is a form of group therapy, wherein the nuclear family is the unit, that has developed during the past three or four decades.

      2. Family therapists view the family as a behavioral system with unique properties. Emotional disturbances of individual members are therefore regarded as outgrowths of conflicts between family members.

      3. One or more therapists deal with an entire family unit during the therapeutic sessions. The goal of treatment is to resolve or reduce the pathogenic conflicts and anxiety within the unit.

   B. Scope

      1. In the past, in certain experimental situations, entire family units were hospitalized so that the genesis of schizophrenia and other emotional disorders could be studied.

      2. Family therapy may be used as the sole treatment, or it may be used in conjunction with other types of therapy.

      3. It has been recommended for marital conflict and child-parent conflicts.

   C. Difficulties

      1. The therapist often finds it difficult to keep the family group intact for sessions. (Siblings resist, parents have to work, and so forth.)

      2. Another difficulty is keeping the focus on the family process and related to the family as a functioning unit rather than shifting to individual members.

V. Somatic therapy

A. Electroconvulsive therapy

1. Since the introduction of the antipsychotic and antidepressant drugs in the late 1950s and early 1960s, the use of electroconvulsive therapy (ECT) as a treatment for schizophrenic disorders has declined, but it remains a treatment for severe affective illness.

2. It is an empirical treatment that relieves symptoms and there is no theory that satisfactorily explains how it acts. Recent neurobiological research suggests that ECT may alter amine metabolism in the central nervous system. (Some researchers have found increased serotonin levels, others have noted a decrease in norepinephrine.) Such a theory seems plausible in light of studies that indicate that catecholamines play a role in affective illnesses.

3. Techniques

   a. Sufficient electrical current is passed through electrodes applied to both temporal areas of the head to produce a grand mal seizure. A series of such treatments is given, the average being six to twelve.

   b. Regressive electroshock, a more intensive course of ECT than the standard one, was employed for a brief period of time about twenty years ago. In this treatment, two or three grand mal convulsions were induced daily until regression had occurred (marked confusion, memory loss, disorganization, lack of verbal spontaneity, slurring of speech, and apathy; in other words, the patient behaved like a helpless infant, with bowel and bladder incontinence and a need to be fed). This was thought to be effective in cases of schizophrenic disorder that had been refractory to other forms of treatment.

   c. In recent years, electrodes have been applied over the non-dominant temporal hemisphere. This unipolar technique is said to produce less post-seizure confusion and memory loss.

   d. Certain medications are given in conjuction with the treatment to minimize apprehension and physical risk. The following drugs are given intravenously.

      (1) Atropine, to reduce salivation and inhibit vagal action

      (2) Succinylcholine chloride ("anectine"), to modify the muscular contractions of the convulsive seizures

      (3) Sedatives, usually pentothal sodium or brevital to put the patient to sleep just prior to the treatment. (Some

physicians use oral barbiturates instead of intravenous pentothal prior to the treatment.) Thus, the patient is put under light general anesthesia for a brief period of time.

e. During the procedure, the patient receives oxygen under pressure.

4. Indications

a. According to a task force of the American Psychiatric Association,

(1) ECT is an effective treatment for—

(a) Severe depression, when the risk of suicide is high, the patient is not taking adequate food or fluids, and when the use of drugs or other therapy is very risky or will take an unacceptably long time.

(b) Severe psychoses characterized by behavior that threatens the safety and well-being of the patient or others, that cannot be controlled by drugs or other means, or for which drugs cannot be employed because of adverse reactions or because of the risk entailed.

(c) Severe catatonia that has not responded to drugs, when the patient is not taking food or fluids, or when drug or other therapy entails unacceptable risk.

(d) Severe mania, when the use of drug therapy entails unacceptable risk or when coexisting medical problems (e.g., recent myocardial infarction) either require prompt resolution of the mania or make the use of drug therapy unacceptable.

(2) ECT is probably effective for—

(a) Depressions, particularly those characterized by vegetative or endogenous symptoms, that have not responded satisfactorily to an adequate course of therapy with antidepressant drugs.

(b) Depressions, particularly those with vegetative or endogenous elements, when drug therapy is contraindicated.

(c) Psychoses, particularly those with an endogenous affective component, that have not responded to an adequate trial of antipsychotic drugs or when drugs cannot be used because of adverse reactions.

        d. It is important to remember that ECT does not insure against relapse.

    5. Contraindications

        a. The physical risk is extremely small, particularly when given with the medications listed under Techniques on p. 269.

        b. There are many physical conditions that were thought to increase the risk of the treatment but, as experience with ECT has increased, the number of physical conditions that contraindicate it has dwindled to a bare minimum (e.g., the presence of a brain tumor with its accompanying increased intracranial pressure; an acute myocardial infarction; abdominal aneurysm).

        c. Cases must be judged individually, however, weighing the possibility of psychiatric recovery against the possible physical risk.

B. Psychosurgery

    1. This treatment dates back to Moniz, who, in 1936, operated on the frontal lobes of the brain to relieve various symptoms of mental illness.

    2. Various procedures are directed at selected areas of the brain, depending upon the type of disabling symptoms present.

    3. Indications

        a. Patients for whom psychosurgery has been recommended generally have had crippling mental disorders (usually crippling obsessive-compulsive disorder) that have not responded to adequate trials of other treatment modalities and that have a poor prognosis.

        b. The results of modern surgery on such carefully selected cases vary with the series; in general, more than 50 percent of the patients show major improvement and a few are made worse by the procedure.

        c. It should be kept in mind that psychosurgery is radical therapy and is used only as a last resort when other methods have failed.

        d. It is performed infrequently in the United States at the present time.

    4. Although this is a radical treatment, it would be premature to abandon it until further evaluation has been made.

VI. Pharmacotherapy (chemotherapy)

A. Principles of psychopharmacology

    1. It is assumed, in the treatment of psychiatric disorders by pharmacotherapy, that the effectiveness of the drug is achieved by action on the central nervous system; in turn, it is implied that at least some psychiatric disorders, especially psychoses, involve defective functioning of the central nervous system.

2. The nervous system can be influenced in many ways, but direct effects are mediated by substances termed *neuroregulators*. These are divided into two categories.
    a. *Neurotransmitters* act at the synapses, where communication among neurons occurs.
    b. *Neuromodulators* act to amplify or dampen the degree and duration of neurotransmitter action, thus providing for a fine tuning of nervous system activity.
3. Sequence of neurotransmitter activity
    a. Neurotransmitters are synthesized and stored within neurons.
    b. Release of neurotransmitters occurs when neurons are stimulated to the point of "firing."
    c. Neurotransmitter substances in the synapse are inactivated by metabolic processes and by reabsorption into the neuron.
    d. Some neurotransmitters stimulate other neurons; others inhibit the neurons they affect.
    e. The synthesis and inactivation of neurotransmitters are complex chemical processes that can be influenced by other substances, including neuroactive drugs that may stimulate the release of neurotransmitters or may block the synthesis, release, synaptic activity, or inactivation of neurotransmitters.
4. Examples of neuroregulators
    a. Several neurotransmitter substances have been identified and established as active in the central nervous system, and others are under investigation.
    b. The neurotransmitters about which most is known are
        (1) Acetycholine (ACh)
        (2) Norepinephrine (NE)
        (3) Dopamine (DA)
        (4) Serotonin (5HT)
        (5) Gamma Amino Butyric Acid (GABA)
    c. The neuroregulatory role of some hormones and polypeptides is being vigorously investigated. Special attention is being given to endorphins and enkephalins (opioid peptides), which appear to modulate response to pain.
5. Current biochemical hypotheses
    a. The biogenic amines are the neurotransmitters that have been implicated as having roles in schizophrenia and affective disorders.
    b. The biogenic amines include (1) serotonin, which is an indoleamine; and (2) norepinephrine and dopamine, which are catecholamines.

c. The biogenic amines theory of depression
   (1) Depression is assumed to reflect a reduced effective level of biogenic amines in brain systems.
   (2) Reserpine is a drug that reduces the level of serotonin, norepinephrine, and dopamine in patients and, in some cases, produces an accompanying clinical depression.
   (3) The major category of antidepressants, the tricyclics, block the "re-uptake" of biogenic amine neurotransmitters from synapses, thus increasing the concentration of the neurotransmitters in the synapses.
   (4) Pharmacological studies have suggested that some depressions may be related to a norepinephrine deficiency, and some others to a serotonin deficiency.
d. The dopamine theory of schizophrenia
   (1) Schizophrenia is assumed to reflect a defect in dopamine-mediated brain systems.
   (2) Amphetamine, which stimulates the release of catecholamines, can produce, in some persons, psychotic symptoms that resemble schizophrenia, and it can also exacerbate psychotic symptoms in acute schizophrenia.
   (3) The class of antipsychotics, the phenothiazines, most effective in treating schizophrenic symptoms act to inhibit or block dopamine mediated transmission.
e. No current biochemical hypothesis is free from conflicting findings and internal contradictions, but the combination of precise diagnosis, pharmacological analysis of drug effects, and investigation of the operation of neuroregulators will extend our knowledge of the nervous system correlates of the psychoses.

B. Psychotropic drugs
   1. History
      a. Rauwolfia derivatives have been used for centuries in India for many illnesses, including mental illness.
      b. At one time, bromides were commonly prescribed for the control of tension.
      c. Prior to the introduction of the "minor tranquilizers," the barbituates were the standard sedatives and hypnotics.
      d. Lithium was first used in Australia in 1949, but it was not accepted into American practice until 1970 because of reports of the severe intoxication and death of patients who used uncontrolled amounts of lithium chloride as a salt substitute.
      e. Tricyclic antidepressants were introduced in the 1950s.
      f. Meprobamate was introduced in 1954.

C. The psychotropic, or psychotherapeutic, drugs include
   1. Antipsychotic agents
   2. Antidepressant agents
   3. Antianxiety agents
   4. Lithium carbonate
D. Antipsychotic agents
   1. There are a large number of these agents, whose effects are characterized more by their similarity than by their differences.
      a. They produce emotional calmness and mental relaxation.
      b. They effectively control symptoms of both acutely and chronically disturbed psychotic patients.
      c. They are capable of producing the reversible "extrapyramidal syndrome" (rigidity, tremors, drooling).
      d. Although they produce a relatively high incidence of annoying side reactions, the reactions are not dangerous.
      e. They create little, if any, habituation or dependency.
      f. They have revolutionized the pattern of treating psychiatric patients. With the advent of the antipsychotic agents, most psychotic patients can be managed with reduced periods of hospitalization or as outpatients.
   2. Indications
      a. They are more efficacious for patients with acute illness and the best prognosis.
      b. The symptoms that respond best to these agents include tension, hyperactivity, hostility, combativeness, negativism, acute delusions, hallucinations, poor self-care, anorexia and, sometimes, seclusiveness.
   3. Toxicity and side reactions
      a. In general, these agents are very safe.
      b. Side effects include certain mild anticholinergic autonomic effects (e.g., dry mouth and blurred vision; feelings of sluggishness); the extrapyramidal syndrome (Parkinson's syndrome); occasionally acute dystonia (including chronic contractions of muscles in the neck, mouth, tongue, and "restless legs").
      c. A late-appearing extrapyramidal syndrome, tardive dyskinesia, occurs occasionally (choreiform, tic-like, involuntary or semi-voluntary muscular movements, classically involving the tongue, face, and neck muscles.)
   4. Types of antipsychotic agents
      a. Among the commonly used antipsychotic agents are
         (1) Phenothiazines
            (a) Aliphatic
               These are chlorpromazine (Thorazine) and triflupromazine (Vesprin)

(b) Piperdines

These are mesoridazine (Serentil); piperaceta-
zine (Quide); and thioridazine (Mellaril)
(c) Piperazines

These are acetophenazine (Tindal); butapera-
zine (Repoise); carphenazine (Proketazine); flu-
phenazine (Prolixin and Permitil); perphenazine
(Trilafon); and trifluoperazine (Stelazine).
(2) Thioxanthenes
(a) Chlorporthixene (Taractan)
(b) Thiothixene (Navane)
(3) Dibenzazepines
(a) Loxapine (Loxitane, Daxolin)
(b) Clozapine (Leponex, experimental)
(4) Butyrophenones, i.e., Haloperidol (Haldol)
(5) Indolones, i.e., molindone (Moban, Lidone)
b. The rauwolfia alkaloids, forms of reserpine (e.g., serpasil)
are now rarely used for the treatment of psychotic disorders.
E. Antidepressant agents
1. There are three types of antidepressant agents.
a. Stimulants
c. Monoamine oxidase inhibitors (MAOI)
b. Tricyclic antidepressants
2. Stimulants
a. Stimulants, for example, dextroamphetamines (Dexedrine);
methamphetamines (Methedrine and Desoxyn); and methylphenidate (Ritalin) have little if any place in the current
treatment of serious depressive disorders.
b. However, Ritalin is often prescribed for *mild* depressions.
3. Tricyclic antidepressants
a. These are the most commonly employed agents in the treatment of depression.
b. They act by blocking the neuronal uptake of amines into
the presynaptic nerve endings (see Principles of psychopharmacology at the beginning of this section).
c. The overall improvement they achieve is about 70 percent.
d. Among the list of the tricylic antidepressent agents that
follows, there are more similarities than differences.
(1) Amtriptyline (Elavil, Endep)
(2) Desipramine (Norpramin, Pertofrane)
(3) Doxepin (Sinequan, Adapin)
(4) Imipramine (Tofranil, also available in generic form)
(5) Nortriptyline (Aventyl, Pamelor)
(6) Protriptyline (Vivactil)

4. Monamine oxidase inhibitors
    a. When tricyclic antidepressants have not produced remission, these become the next choice.
    b. The MAO inhibitors still in use are
        (1) Tranylcypromine (Parnate)
        (2) Phenelzine (Nardil)
5. Toxicity and side reactions of antidepressant agents
    a. The changeover to MAO inhibitors after using tricyclics requires a waiting period of one to two weeks in order to avoid the rare but serious reactions that may ensue (e.g., hyperprexia, convulsions).
    b. The tricyclic and MAO inhibitors often have the anticholinergic effects listed under the antipsychotic agents (dry mouth, sweating, blurred vision, etc.)
    c. A small caution for people who are using Parnate and Nardil is that they must avoid foods that have a high tyrmine content and certain other drugs which contain sympathominetic amines, since there is danger of a "hypertensive crisis."
F. Antianxiety agents
    1. Characteristics of antianxiety agents
        a. They produce calmness and relaxation, but of a different quality than the antipsychotic agents.
        b. They are not useful in ameliorating disturbed psychotic reactions but are helpful in relieving anxiety and tension.
        c. They have little effect on autonomic functions (except for the antihistamines).
        d. All have depressant effects on the central nervous system.
        e. Many also have muscle relaxant and anti-convulsant properties.
    2. Toxicity and side reactions
        a. They do not produce extrapyramidal phenomena.
        b. Annoying side reactions are relatively rare.
        c. There is some risk of abuse, habituation, and addiction with these agents.
    3. Indications
        a. The chief use of antianxiety agents is in the treatment of relatively transient forms of anxiety and fearfulness.
        b. They are also commonly used as pre-operative sedatives and in the management of pain syndromes, especially those accompanied by muscular tension.
    4. List of commonly used antianxiety agents
        a. Meprobamate (Equanil, Miltown) is listed here because of its historical importance. It is not commonly used at present.

b. Antihistamines
  (1) Diphenylmethane (Benadryl)
  (2) Hydroxyzine (Atarax)
  (3) Hydroxyzine pamoate (Vistaril)
c. Benzodiazepine derivatives
  (1) Chlordiazepoxide (Librium)
  (2) Diazepam (Valium)
    (a) This has become the most commonly prescribed of all drugs.
    (b) It has also become a popularly abused drug because it acts rapidly and tends to produce euphoria.
  (3) Oxazepam (Serax)
  (4) Lorezapam (Ativan)
  (5) Clorazepate dipotassium (Tranxene)
  (6) Clorazepate monopotassium (Azene)
  (7) Prazepam (Verstran)
G. Lithium carbonate
  1. Forms of lithium carbonate are Lithane, Lithonate, and Eskalith.
  2. The mechanism of action of lithium in affective disorders is not clearly understood.
  3. Indications
    a. Acute mania and hypomania
    b. Prophylactically, to prevent recurrent attacks of mania in bipolar affective disorders.
    c. Thought by some to be helpful in "schizoaffective disorder."
  4. Summary
    a. Although lithium is a specific form of treatment for manic and hypomanic episodes, it is often necessary, because there is a delay in its action, to use another antipsychotic agent initially (e.g., Chlorpromazine, Thioridazine, or Haloperidol) to control the disturbed behavior.
    b. Its main limitation is the narrowness between the therapeutic range and the toxic range.
    c. It seems most promising because of its prophylactic effect in reducing the frequency and severity of episodes in bipolar disorders.

VII. Management therapy

There are a number of activities, apart from formal psychotherapy, group psychotherapy, somatic therapy, and chemotherapy, that have psychotherapeutic value. Among them are attitude therapy, occupational therapy, and therapeutic recreation.

A. Attitude therapy

Attitude therapy is an attempt to prescribe the attitude that the entire staff and personnel will assume toward a patient. Some examples follow.

1. An attitude of indifference is often effective in the management of certain conversion symptoms.
2. A firm but nonpunitive attitude is often necessary in managing antisocial behavior.
3. Confrontation and prescription of consequences are often useful in managing acting-out adolescents.
4. A reassuring attitude may be necessary in the management of patients who are anxious and fearful.

B. Occupational therapy

There are many activities and situations which the occupational therapist utilizes psychotherapeutically to meet the individual's needs and provide a vehicle for personal change and growth. Some examples follow.

1. The use of the punching bag to relieve hostile and aggressive feelings.
2. Utilizing creative media such as clay and painting to express creative needs and to portray feelings and conflicts that may be difficult to express verbally.
3. Improving living skills (e.g., self-care, cooking, communication, transportation) through education and practice.
4. The use of gross motor activities (e.g., sawing, sanding, weaving rugs) to provide appropriate outlets for anger, hostility, and tension.

C. Therapeutic recreation

Numerous recreational activities are used therapeutically to promote personal change and growth. Some examples follow.

1. The use of the punching bag or racket ball to relieve hostile and aggressive feelings.
2. The use of team activities for the development of leadership, cooperation, and social interaction.
3. Leisure education to aid in the development of new interests and to provide balance in the individual's daily life.

D. Psychodrama

In this form of therapy, patients dramatize their emotional problems in group settings. A leading proponent of this therapy is Moreno.

VIII. Behavior therapy

Behavior therapy has a specific meaning when used by some writers, but it will be used here as a general term that refers to all therapy that is derived from principles of learning (see the chapter, "Behavioral Concepts," written by Shirley H. Mink, Ph.D. and Walter D. Mink, Ph.D.).

A. Background
   1. Pavlov, late in his career, attempted to give an account of human psychiatric disorders in terms of excitation and inhibition, the concepts that had so successfully accounted for data from his animal laboratory. His clinical interpretations were less successful, but he did stimulate other experimental scientists of learning to apply their analyses to clinical disorders.
   2. Watson (1920) and Jones (1924) demonstrated how a focal fear or phobia could be learned and extinguished by classical conditioning, but these demonstrations had no significant impact on the practice or theory of clinical psychiatry.
   3. Psychologists working with children with poor "habits" (e.g., nailbiting, bed-wetting, temper tantrums) during the 1920s and 1930s developed practical techniques that are now viewed as forms of behavior therapy (Dunlop, 1930).
   4. Learning theorists such as O. H. Mowrer (1950), Neal Miller and John Dollard (1950), attempted to interpret psychoanalytic theory and therapy in terms of the systematic learning theory of Clark Hull (1943); their writings renewed the interest of some experimental psychologists in psychiatric problems.
   5. B. F. Skinner and his student, Ogden Lindsley (1954), applied operant analysis of learning to the behavior of schizophrenics, and this incursion into the realm of psychiatric disorder was rapidly followed by the application of the same methods to treatment or, in operant conditioning terminology, behavior modification.
   6. The publication by Joseph Wolpe in 1958 of his book *Psychotherapy by Reciprocal Inhibition* attracted widespread attention to developments in therapy in several countries and signaled the beginning of the modern era of behavior therapy.
   7. Hans Eysenck (1958) encouraged a systematic approach to the theory and practice of behavior therapy by emphasizing the main points of difference from traditional psychotherapy.

B. General principles
   1. Behavior therapy can be defined as the modification of responses through the application of experimentally established principles of learning.
   2. Maladaptive behavior is viewed as either deficient or excessive. Thus, therapy involves increasing the incidence of appropriate behavior and decreasing behavior that is inappropriate in frequency, duration, or place of occurrence.

3. Maladaptive responses may be covert as well as overt. Thus, such traditional cognitive symptoms as hallucinations, delusions, and fantasies are not, in principle, recalcitrant to behavior therapy.
4. Psychiatric disorders are viewed primarily, though not exclusively, as the result of faulty learning.
5. Treatment is directed toward the removal of the inappropriate behavior (symptoms) and toward learning new, more effective patterns of behavior.
6. Emphasis in treatment is placed particularly on the social environment as a source of stimuli that support symptoms but that can also support changes in behavior.
7. The experimental study of learning and the clinical practice of behavior therapy are viewed as mutually supporting activities that together can contribute to a unified understanding of learned behavior.

C. Types of behavior therapy

There are many variants of behavior therapy, but the examples that follow typify the most widely used techniques.

1. Systematic desensitization
    a. This technique was developed by Joseph Wolpe as a means of associating anxiety-eliciting stimuli with relaxation.
    b. Since anxiety and relaxation are incompatible reactions, the increase in the strength of relaxation responses will inhibit the anxious responses to the same stimuli.
    c. Wolpe's approach consists of three stages.
        (1) Relaxation training similar to the procedures introduced by Jacobson in 1938, in which the subject is taught to identify and control localized tension and relaxation of muscle groups.
        (2) Construction of hierarchies of anxiety-producing stimuli by the subject; these threatening stimuli or events in the subject's life are ranked by the reactions they produce, from the weakest to strongest.
        (3) Desensitization proper. The subject, in a deep state of relaxation, is presented with a stimulus from the weak end of the hierarchy and then with successively stronger ones as he or she is able to maintain relaxation.
    d. Variations of this "gradual-approach" method have been used to rehearse adequate behavior in an anxiety-inhibiting context (e.g., assertiveness training).

2. Aversion therapy
   a. This is the oldest of the three procedures outlined in this section, but it was used for many years with little systematic attention to the principles of learning that were applied.
   b. This therapy is based on straightforward classical (Pavlovian) conditioning procedures. Stimuli are associated with some strong, unacceptable responses such as nausea, pain, or extreme disgust.
   c. The noxious stimuli that are used to produce the response of aversion may be chemical (e.g., apomorphine), electrical, or visual (including imaginal).
   d. Aversion therapy has most often been used in the treatment of habitual excesses (e.g., overuse of alcohol) and compulsive unacceptable or criminal social behavior (e.g., shoplifting, exhibitionism).
   e. Considerable controversy has been generated both about the effectiveness of aversion therapy and the social appropriateness of aversive control of socially deviant behavior. (The novel and movie *A Clockwork Orange* provide examples of the social concern about aversive control of behavior.)
   f. Both operant conditioning analyses of the effect of aversive stimuli and the exploration of the effect of aversive imagery are attempts to find less unpleasant and more socially acceptable alternatives to aversion therapy.

3. Behavior modification
   a. *Behavior modification* is conducted by the application of operant conditioning principles to the interpretation and management of behavior problems.
   b. The basic principle of behavior modification is the control of the reinforcing consequences of behavior. *Reinforcing consequences* range from physical reinforcers (e.g., food) to social reinforcers (e.g., approval, tokens of exchange).
   c. Behavior modification has been used in a variety of institutional settings and on a great variety of problems. Striking examples include language training of autistic children, self-care training of intellectually retarded children and adults, and socialization of regressed psychotic patients.
   d. Some wards of psychiatric hospitals and some entire institutions are managed according to operant conditioning principles in a "token economy." That is, appropriate changes in behavior are rewarded with tokens that can be exchanged for food, activities, and privileges.

e. Self-regulation techniques, by which patients learn to distinguish the environmental stimuli that evoke their maladaptive behavior and to manage their own reinforcing consequences, have grown in popularity among behavior therapists and have become a significant part of the popular literature of self-treatment.

f. Biofeedback techniques are a form of self-regulation based on operant methods. The subjects monitor their own physiological processes (muscle tension, brain waves) and, using the information they receive (feedback), learn to control them within limits.

g. Behavior modification is the most active, rapidly expanding, and enthusiastically professed learning approach to therapy.

4. Cognitive behavior therapy

a. Early approaches to behavior therapy minimized or excluded from consideration such cognitive or mental variables as images, thoughts, expectations, or beliefs.

b. Many practitioners of behavior therapy, however, now assume that self-statements provide a basis for inferences about cognition and accept the idea that the beliefs and expectations that mediate much maladaptive behavior can be modified by behavior therapy.

c. The approach of Albert Ellis, rational-emotive therapy, emphasizes change in maladaptive behavior by the therapist confronting patients with their irrational beliefs and helping them to restructure their behavior by adapting a more rational set of beliefs by which they can live.

d. Aaron Beck, in his recommendations for the treatment of depression, likewise assigns major importance to correcting the faulty thinking that produces a negative bias toward oneself and negative expectations about the reinforcement available in one's present or future environment.

e. To many practitioners, however, the integration of cognitive and behavior treatment modes is controversial because they believe that concern with inferred mental states will reduce the effectiveness of direct manipulation of the environment.

5. Evaluation

a. While behavior therapy was initially developed for and applied in the treatment of phobias and compulsions, it does not appear to be limited to reactions (symptoms) that obviously fit a learning interpretation.

b. Since the emphasis in treatment is on modification of symp-
      toms, the question of substitution has been raised by some
      critics (i.e., the removal of one symptom may lead to
      another if the underlying cause is not also treated). How-
      ever, according to proponents of the therapy, substitution
      does not usually occur.
   c. Some enthusiastic supporters of behavior therapy, such as
      Hans Eysenck, claim that their evaluations show behavior
      therapy to be clearly superior to other forms of psycho-
      therapy, particularly psychoanalysis.
   d. More moderate and well-controlled evaluations indicate
      that behavior therapy is useful, that it is at least as effective
      as traditional psychotherapy, and that it may have partic-
      ular benefits.
   e. Since experimental investigations of learning and clinical
      applications of behavior therapy make use of similar con-
      cepts and sources of evidence, a consistent association
      between laboratory and clinic is maintained in this
      approach to treatment.

IX. Humanistic therapy

A number of therapeutic approaches characterized by their phenomenological or existential assumptions about human experiences or by
their opposition to traditional psychoanalysis or behavior therapy have
come to be loosely referred to as "humanistic" therapy. While *humanistic* is a word with many connotations, it is used here merely as a
conventional label for these approaches.

A. Principles
   1. A person's world is a product of individual perceptions. There-
      fore, what one says about one's personal world should be
      accepted as subjective truth.
   2. Each person is unique. Therefore, individual dignity must not
      be affronted by the attempt to label, categorize, or reduce a
      person to some set of generalizations about human character
      or behavior.
   3. Individuals are processes, rather than products of influences.
      Thus, each person has, in principle, the capacity to realize his
      or her potentialities and to live the life suited to those poten-
      tialities.
   4. Individuals are free, capable of choice, and responsible for the
      choices, fulfilling or unfulfilling, that they make.
   5. The goals of treatment are those that the patients choose freely
      and that are congruent with their understanding of themselves
      and their interests.

6. The role of the therapist is to provide a supportive, understanding, and accepting context for the exploration of opportunities for personal growth and development.

B. Variants

There are many variants of humanistic therapy, both individual and group. The following have achieved wide recognition.

1. Client-centered therapy
    a. The chief proponent of client-centered therapy is Carl Rogers.
    b. Rogers believes that there is a strong innate tendency to develop and realize one's potentialities. Nevertheless, a person may adopt a set of values or attitudes that limits experience or blocks development.
    c. The therapist offers total acceptance, which is the necessary condition of change.
    d. The therapist uses techniques of recognition and clarification of the client's feelings, and encourages honesty in communication.
    e. In a therapeutic context of this kind, the client can reassess his or her self-perceptions and make constructive choices.

2. Existential analysis
    a. Exponents include Medard Boss, Viktor Frankl, and Rollo May.
    b. They believe that people define themselves in terms of interpersonal relationships and that the relationships must be honest and open (authentic) to give existence its value and meaning.
    c. Patients' symptoms reflect evasions of responsibility for their own choices, for their dysphoria, or for their unstable or incoherent set of values (meaninglessness).
    d. The therapist encourages the patient to accept responsibility for symptoms as self-chosen and to decide on ways of dealing with life that are active, authentic, and meaningful.
    e. Since individuals (and therapists) are unique, no particular techniques and procedures can be formulated as general principles.

3. Gestalt therapy
    a. Fritz Perls is the leading proponent of gestalt therapy.
    b. Disordered behavior is viewed as the result of unresolved past conflicts, but its resolution occurs in the action and decisions of the here-and-now.
    c. Emphasis is placed on the identification and acceptance of one's needs and one's personal responsibility for meeting them by selecting effective strategies.

d. Gestalt therapy is more technique-oriented than the other two humanistic therapies, using reenactment of dreams, role-played conversations with one's own feelings or with other persons or objects, cathartic "acting-out," and interpersonal confrontation in groups.

　　e. The gestalt therapist is also more direct and manipulative in treatment sessions, but the patient is responsible for defining the changes to be made and for exploring change.

　　f. The goal of gestalt therapy (the German word *gestalt* means "whole") is the unification of feeling and action into a new configuration of decisive and fulfilling experience.

C. Evaluation

　1. There has been little evaluation of humanistic therapy by practitioners. Evaluation is viewed as a violation of the humanistic emphasis on the uniqueness and integrity of the individual. Carl Rogers's research program is an exception.

　2. Concern with individual responsibility and choice is not the exclusive domain of humanistic approaches, though these approaches have led to a re-evaluation of the role of self-determination in other types of therapy.

　3. It is doubtful that any therapeutic situation is as free from the therapist's influence as the humanistic therapists claim theirs are.

　4. The humanistic perspective is viewed by some critics as reflecting an unscientific and even antiscientific approach to the understanding and treatment of human problems.

　5. Nevertheless, humanistic therapy has achieved popular acceptance and has had a major role in the development of alternatives to traditional psychiatric and psychological treatment.

References

American Psychiatric Association. *A Psychiatric Glossary*. 5th ed. Washington, D. C., 1980.

————. *Electroconvulsive Therapy*, Task Report No. 14. Washington, D. C., 1978.

Baldessarini, R. J. *Chemotherapy in Psychiatry*. Cambridge: Harvard University Press, 1977.

Barchas, J. D., Bergen, P. A., Ciaranello, R. D., and Elliott, G. R., eds. *Psychopharmacology: From Theory to Practice*. New York: Oxford University Press, 1977.

Beck, A. T. *Depression: Clinical, Experimental, and Theoretical Aspects*. New York: Harper & Row, Publishers, 1967.

Benson, W. M., and Schiele, B. C. *Tranquilizing and Antidepressive Drugs*. Springfield, Ill.: Charles C Thomas, Publisher, 1962.

Bergin, A. E., and Garfield, S. L. *Handbook of Psychotherapy and Behavior Change: An Empirical Analysis*. New York: John Wiley & Sons, 1971.

Boss, M. *Psychoanalysis and Daseinsanalysis*. New York: Basic Books, Inc., Publishers, 1967.

Calhoun, J. F., et al. *Abnormal Psychology: Current Perspectives*. 2d ed. New York: CRM/Random House, 1977.

Dollard, J., and Miller, N. E. *Personality and Psychotherapy*. New York: McGraw-Hill, 1950.

Dunlap, K. *Habits: Their Making and Unmaking.* New York: Liverwright, 1932.

Eyesenck, H. J. "The Effects of Psychotherapy: An Evaluation." *Journal of Consulting Psychology* 16(1952): 319-324.

Ellis, A. *Reason and Emotion in Psychotherapy.* New York: Lyle Stuart, Inc., 1962.

Frankl, V. E. *Psychotherapy and Existentialism.* New York: Washington Square Press, 1967.

Freedman, A. M.; Kaplan, H. I.; and Sadock, B. J. *Modern Synopsis of Comprehensive Textbook of Psychiatry.* Vol. 2. 2d ed. Baltimore: Williams & Wilkins Company, 1976, chaps. 29, 30, 31.

Jacobson, E. *Progressive Relaxation.* Chicago: University of Chicago Press, 1938.

Kalinowsky, L. B., and Hoch, P. H. *Somatic Treatment in Psychiatry.* New York: Grune & Stratton, 1961.

Kolb, L. C. *Modern Clinical Psychiatry.* 9th ed. Philadelphia: W. B. Saunders Company, chaps. 1977, 30, 32, 33.

Leitenberg, H., ed. *Handbook of Behavior Modification and Behavior Therapy.* Englewood Cliffs, N. J.: Prentice-Hall, 1976.

Lindsley, O. R. "Operant Conditioning Methods Applied to Research in Chronic Schizophrenia." *Psychiatric Research Reports* 5(1956): 118–139.

Lunzer, R. G. Personal communication, February 1969.

May, R. "Contributions of Existential Psychotherapy." In R. May, F. Angel, and H. F. Ellenberger (Eds.), *Existence: A New Dimension in Psychiatry and Psychology.* Basic Books, Inc., Publishers, 1958 a).

Mowrer, O. H. *Learning Theory and Personality Dynamics.* New York: The Ronald Press Company, 1950.

Nicholi, A. M., Jr., ed. *The Harvard Guide to Modern Psychiatry.* Cambridge: Belknap Press of Harvard University Press, 1978, chaps. 17, 18, 21, 22.

Perls, F. S. *Four Lectures.* In J. Fagan and I. L. Shepherd, Eds., *Gestalt Therapy Now: Therapy, Techniques, Applications.* Palo Alto, Calif.: Science and Behavior Books, 1970.

Rogers, C. R. *On Becoming a Person.* Boston: Houghton Mifflin Company, 1961.

Stuart, R. B., ed. *Behavioral Self-Management: Strategies, Techniques and Outcomes.* New York: Bunner/Mazel, 1977.

Wolpe, J. *Psychotherapy by Reciprocal Inhibition.* Stanford, Calif.: Stanford University Press, 1958.

Glossary

Acrophobia   Fear of heights.

Active influence   The psychotic belief that one controls others.

Actual self   The sum total of an individual's experiences.

Adjustment disorder   A maladaptive reaction to an identifiable life event or circumstance that is not merely an exacerbation of one of the mental disorders and that is expected to remit, if and when the stressor ceases.

Affect   Mood or feeling tone.

Affective disorder   A mental disorder in which the fundamental disturbance is in the mood.

Agitation   A state of restlessness and uneasiness, often characterized by such muscular manifestations as motor restlessness; mental perturbation.

Agoraphobia   A phobic disorder in which the predominant disturbance is an irrational fear of leaving the familiar setting of the home.

Alcohol amnestic syndrome (Korsakoff's syndrome)   Irreversible amnesia associated with disorientation, confabulation, and peripheral neuropathy.

Alcohol hallucinosis   Hallucinosis that persists after a person has recovered from the symptoms of alcohol withdrawal and is no longer drinking.

Alcohol idiosyncratic intoxication (pathological intoxication)   Overreaction to minimal amounts of alcohol, less than sufficient to cause intoxication in most people.

Alcohol intoxication   Simple intoxication in which there is slurred speech, incoordination, unsteady gait, and impairment of memory.

Alcohol withdrawal   The development of withdrawal symptoms shortly after not drinking for several days or longer.

Alcohol withdrawal delirium   An acute psychotic episode occurring within one week after the cessation or reduction of heavy alcohol intake, characterized by delirium, coarse tremors, and perceptual disturbances, including illusions and frightening visual hallucinations that usually become more intense in the dark.

Alcoholics   Those excessive drinkers whose dependence upon alcohol has attained such a degree that it causes a noticeable mental disturbance or interferes with the drinkers' bodily and mental health, their interpersonal relationships, or their smooth and economic functioning.

Alcoholics Anonymous (AA)   An informal, worldwide fellowship of groups of alcoholics who help each other to stay sober and to remain abstinent.

Alcoholism   A disorder characterized by excessive use of alcohol to the point of habituation, overdependence, or addiction.

Algolagnia, active   Sadism.

Algolagnia, passive   Masochism.

Alzheimer's disease   A presenile diffuse, degenerative, organic brain disease.

Ambivalence   The coexistence of two opposing feelings toward the same individual or object; feelings may be conscious, unconscious, or partly both.

Amnesia   A pathological loss of memory.

Amnesia, anterograde   Loss of memory of events that occur after a particular time.

Amnesia, retrograde   Loss of memory of events that occurred before a particular time.

Amnestic syndrome   Short-term, but not immediate, memory disturbance, in the absence of dementia or delirium.

Amphetamine   A drug that stimulates release of catecholamines and may also produce in some persons psychotic symptoms that resemble schizophrenia; may exacerbate psychotic symptoms in acute schizophrenia.

Anaclitic   Dependency on others; for example, the dependent relationship the infant has with its mother.

Anal phase   The period from the eighteenth month until the end of the third year in which the infant's attention is centered on excretory functions.

Analgesia   Diminished sense of pain.

Anancastic personality (anal character)   An individual who needs to feel in control of himself or herself and of the environment.

Anesthesia   Absence of feeling.

Anima   The true inner self or soul.

Anima   The female component of the male personality.

Animus   The masculine component of the female personality.

Anorexia nervosa   A syndrome marked by severe and prolonged inability to eat, with marked weight loss, amenorrhea (absence of menstrual discharge) or impotence, and other symptoms resulting from emotional conflict and biological changes.

Antisocial personality disorder   A disorder with a history of continuous and chronic antisocial behavior in which the rights of others are violated; onset occurs before age fifteen; the persistence of antisocial behavior after the age of fifteen into adult life; and failure to sustain a good job performance over a period of several years.

Anxiety   A diffuse, unpleasant uneasiness, apprehension, or fearfulness stemming from anticipated danger, the source of which is unidentifiable.

Anxiety disorder   Some form of anxiety in which either the most prominent disturbance in the clinical picture, as in panic disorder or anxiety, is experienced because the individual tries to resist succumbing to other symptoms, as in avoidance of a dreaded object or situation (in a phobic disorder) and obsessions or compulsions (in an obsessive compulsive disorder).

Apathy   Lack of feeling, emotion, interest, or concern; impassiveness or unfeelingness.

Aphonia   Inability to produce normal speech.

Apperception   A mental act in which the mind becomes aware or has knowledge of itself as it perceives.

Aptitude tests   Tests that measure a variety of special aptitudes and abilities.

Asexual   A person who denies ever having strong sexual feelings.

Asthma   An allergic disorder with dyspnea (labored respiration) and wheezing due to bronchial obstruction resulting from bronchial spasm, bronchial edema, and mucus plugs.

Atropine   A drug used to reduce salivation and inhibit action of the vagal nerve.

Attention   Maintenance of focused consciousness on the salient characteristics of the environment.

Attitude therapy   An attempt to prescribe the attitude that a mental health staff and personnel will assume toward a patient.

Atypical paranoid disorder (paranoid state)   An ill-defined group of reactions characterized by paranoid delusions that lack the logical systematization seen in paranoia but do not involve the regression, bizarreness, and deterioration found in paranoid schizophrenia. This is a residual category for paranoid disorders that are not classifiable elsewhere.

Auditory illusions   Mistaken interpretation of sounds.

Autism   Fantasy and daydreaming that substitutes for reality; a persistent overindulgence in fantasy.

Autochthonous ideas   Ideas originating within the psyche without external stimuli.

Automatism   Unconsciously directed automatic, repetitive, and symbolic behavior observed in schizophrenic, convulsive, and dissociative disorders.

Aversion therapy   A form of therapy based on straightforward classical (Pavlovian) conditioning procedures.

Avoidant personality disorder   A disorder in which there is hypersensitivity to rejection and unwillingness to enter into relationships unless given unusually strong guarantees of uncritical acceptance; social withdrawal, with a desire for affection and acceptance; low self-esteem.

Behavior modification   The application of operant conditioning principles to the interpretation and management of behavioral problems.

Behavior therapy   A general term that refers to all therapy that is derived from principles of learning.

Behaviorism   John Watson's definition for the methodological position in psychology.

Biofeedback techniques   A form of self-regulation, based on operant methods, in which subjects monitor their own physiological processes (muscle tension, brain waves) and using the information they received (feedback), learn to control them, within limits.

Bi-polar disorder   Manic-depressive disease.

Birth trauma   Primal anxiety, in response to feelings of helplessness, produced by birth.

Blocking   Difficulty in recalling or interpreting a stream of speech or thought because of emotional forces that are usually conscious.

Blunting of attention   Extreme inattention so that even noxious stimulation may not elicit a response.

Borderline personality disorder   A disorder in which there is instability in a variety of areas, including interpersonal relationships, behavior, mood, and self-image.

Brief reactive psychosis   A psychotic disorder of at least a few hours duration but lasting no more than one week, with a sudden onset immediately following a recognizable stressor that would be expected to evoke significant symptoms of distress in almost all individuals; i.e., loss of a loved one or the psychological trauma of combat.

Bulimia   Increased appetite.

Castration anxiety   Anxiety stemming from the fear of damage to or loss of male genitals.

Catalepsy   A generalized diminished responsiveness or immobility characterized by trance-like states.

Catatonic excitement   A form of schizophrenia characterized by extreme psychomotor agitation; purposeless and stereotyped excited motor activity that is not influenced by external stimuli.

Catatonic posturing   A form of schizophrenia in which there is voluntary assumption of inappropriate or bizarre posture.

Catatonic rigidity   A form of schizophrenia in which patients maintain a rigid posture against efforts to move them.

Catatonic stupor or mutism   A form of schizophrenia characterized by mutism, marked decreased reactivity to the environment, reduction of spontaneous movements and activities.

Cathexis   The process by which the unconscious primitive drives are vested with psychic energy.

Circumstantiality   Incidental or adventitious thinking.

Clang association   A disturbance in thinking in which the sound of a word, rather than its meaning, sets off a new train of thought.

Clarification   A process by which the physician helps patients to understand their feelings and behavior and to gain a clearer picture of reality.

Clouding of consciousness   Impairment of retention, perception, and orientation.

Collective unconscious   Racial or archaic unconsciousness, in which there is an inheritance of primitive racial ideas and impulses.

Coma (stupor)   A state of unawareness and nonreactiveness; profound unconsciousness.

Compensation   A conscious or unconscious attempt to overcome real or fancied inferiorities.

Compulsions   Repetitive and seemingly purposeful behaviors that are performed according to certain rules or in a stereotyped fashion. The behavior is not an end in itself, but is designed to produce or prevent some future event or situation. However, either the activity is not connected in a realistic way with what it is designed to produce or prevent, or may be clearly excessive. The act is performed with a sense of subjective compulsion coupled with a desire to resist the compulsion (at least initially). The individual generally recognizes the senselessness of the behavior (this may not be true for young children) and does not derive pleasure from carrying out the activity, although it provides a release of tension.

Compulsive personality disorder   A disorder in which there is restricted ability to express warm and tender emotions; preoccupation with matters of rules, order, organization, efficiency, and details, with a loss of ability to focus on "the big picture"; insistence that others submit to one's way of doing things; excessive devotion to work and productivity to the exclusion of pleasure; indecisiveness.

Conation   The basic strivings of an individual as expressed in his or her behavior.

Condensation   The contraction of several different ideas into one phrase, forming a collage of thought; the coalition of several concepts into one.

Confabulation   A falsification of memory in which gaps in memory are filled in by imaginary (fabricated) experiences that seem plausible and are recounted in detail.

Confusion   Disorientation in respect to time, place, or person, accompanied by perplexity.

Conscience   The conscious part of superego.

Conscious   The state of being of an individual composed of ideas, feelings, drives, and urges of which the person is aware.

Consciousness   The conscious.

Conversion disorder   A clinical picture in which the predominant disturbance is a loss or alternation of physical functioning that suggests a physical disorder but that is actually a direct expression of psychological conflict or need.

Coping mechanisms   Conscious attempts to control anxiety.

Coprolalia   The compulsive utterance of obscene words.

Coprophagia   A desire to eat feces.

Coprophilia   A pathological sexual interest in excretions.

Cosmic consciousness or illumination   A fabulous sense of joy or well-being, sometimes produced by hallucinogenic drugs.

Counter-cathexis   The opposition of ego energy to id energy.

Countertransference   The therapist's unconscious or conscious emotional reaction to the patient.

Cyclothymic disorder   A disorder characterized by recurring and alternating periods of depression and elation not readily attributable to external circumstances.

Defense mechanisms   Specific, unconscious, intrapsychic adjustments that come into play to resolve emotional conflict and reduce the individual's anxiety.

Defenses   Unconscious ways of dealing with anxiety.

Déjà vu   The sensation that an experience that is really happening for the first time occurred previously.

Delirium   A condition characterized by disturbance in affect, memory, or consciousness.

Delusions   Fixed false beliefs that are not in keeping with the individual's cultural or intellectual level.

Dementia   Organic loss of intellectual function.

Denial   The unconscious disavowal of a thought, feeling, wish, need, or reality that is consciously unacceptable.

Dependent personality disorder   A disorder in which the essential features are getting others to assume responsibility for major areas of one's life;

subordinating one's own needs to rely on oneself; lack of self-confidence; intense discomfort when alone for more than brief periods.

Depersonalization Pervasive feelings of unreality, strangeness, or altered identity or, a sense of estrangement from oneself.

Depersonalization disorder An alteration in the perception or experience of the self so that the feelings of one's own reality is temporarily lost. It can also be defined as a disorder of affect in which the person has feelings of unreality or altered identity.

Depression A feeling of sadness, loneliness, dejection, or hopelessness.

Derailment (disturbance of association) Looseness of association.

Derealization Feeling that the environment has changed.

Deterioration (dementia) The progressive loss of intellectual and emotional functions.

Diasthesis-stress theory A theory that assumes that certain genes or gene combinations give rise to a predisposing (diasthesis) toward a particular disorder.

Disorientation Loss of awareness of one's position in relationship to time, surroundings, or other persons.

Displacement The redirection of an emotion from the original object to a more acceptable substitute.

Dissociation The unconscious detachment of certain behavior from the normal or usual conscious behavior patterns of an individual, which then function alone (compartmentalization).

Dissociative disorder A disorder in which the person has feelings of unreality, altered personality, or altered identity and might deny his or her own existence along with that of his or her environment.

Distractibility A heightened rapid fluctuation of attention so that every new stimulus, regardless of significance, is responded to by rapid shift.

Dizygotic twins Fraternal twins.

Dream state (twilight state) A transient clouding of consciousness of intrapsychic origin during which the person is unaware of reality and behaves violently or opposite to his or her usual pattern.

Dysthymic disorder (depressive neurosis) Mild, intermittent or sustained depression of at least two years duration.

Echolalia The pathological repetition of phrases or words of another person.

Echopraxia The pathological repetition or imitation of movements the subject is observing.

Ecstasy A feeling of intense rapture found in states of depersonalization and certain psychoses, such as schizophrenic disorders.

Ego The part of the personality that meets and interacts with the outside world; the "integrator" or "mediator" of the personality.

Ego-dystonic homosexuality A disorder in which individuals' sexual interests are directed primarily toward people of the same sex and who are either disturbed by, in conflict with, or wish to change their sexual orientation.

Ego-ideal The nonpunitive, positive aspect of the superego.

Ego-libido Libido concentrated on the self; narcissism.

Eidetic imagery Vivid, accurate, and detailed visual after-images; sometimes called photographic memory.

Elation   Marked euphoria, accompanied by increased motor activity.

Electra complex   The Oedipus complex of aggressive feeling in the female.

Electroconvulsive therapy (ECT)   A form of psychiatric treatment in which sufficient electrical current is passed through electrodes applied to both temporal areas of the head to produce a grand mal seizure.

Empathy   The capacity for participating in, or for vicariously experiencing another's feelings, volitions, or ideas.

Endogenous-reactive dichotomy   Subdivision of depression based on whether or not the depression was related to life events (reactive) or seemed to develop "from within" (endogenous).

Environmental modification (environmental manipulation)   The altering of the environment so as to relieve the patient's symptoms and distress.

Eros   The name given to the creative forces; the life instinct.

Erotic delusion   Delusions that may concern infidelity, sexual exploitation, change of sex, or the grandiose idea of being loved by someone else, often a famous person (who must keep secret the love relationship).

Erotomania   Pathological preoccupation with erratic fantasies or activities.

Essential alcoholism   Addictive drinking, compulsive drinking, or alcoholism simplex.

Essential hypertension   *See* Hypertension.

Euphoria   An exaggerated sense of well-being not consistent with reality.

Excitement   The subjective sense of sexual pleasure with accompanying psychological changes.

Exhibitionism   A disorder in which there are repetitive acts of exposing the genitals to an unsuspecting stranger for the purpose of producing sexual excitement.

Experimental neurosis   Pavlov's definition for a disorganization in the behavior of animals who are required to make extremely difficult conditioned discriminations.

Extra-psychic   From outside the environment.

Extroversion   Outwardly directed libido.

Exultation   Intense elation accompanied by grandiose feelings.

Factitious disorders   Factitious (or pseudo; unnatural) conditions that are produced by individuals, under voluntary control and who do not appear goal-directed.

Family therapy   A form of group therapy, in which the nuclear family is the unit, that has developed during the past three or four decades as a direct approach to the mental health of the family as an interacting unit.

Fantasy (phantasy)   Fabricated series of mental pictures or sequences of events; daydreaming.

Fascination (or fixation)   A trance-like state in individuals (e.g., pilots) who are compelled to focus on a given object for long periods of time.

Fausse reconnaissance   A false recognition of the unfamiliar.

Feelings of derealization   Feelings that the environment has changed.

Feelings of estrangement   A sense of detachment from people, the environment, or concepts.

Feelings of unreality   Feelings that one is unreal.

Fetishism   A disorder in which there is use of inanimate objects as the preferred or exclusive method of producing sexual excitement.

Fixation   The arrest of maturation at an immature level of psychosexual development.

Flagellation   Erotic whipping.

Flight of ideas   Skipping from one idea to another in quick succession, without reaching the goal of the thinking.

Fluctuation of attention   A greater than normal variation, sometimes to the point of inability to attend in spite of the attempt to do so.

Free-floating anxiety   Severe, persistent, generalized, and unattached anxiety.

Frottage (frotteurism)   Sexual pleasure obtained from rubbing or pressing against fully clothed members of the opposite sex.

Fugue state   Dissociation, a flight from the immediate environment, characterized by an inability to remember what is happening.

Gender-identity disorders   Disorders characterized by an individual's feeling of discomfort and inappropriateness about his or her anatomic sex and by persistent behavior generally associated with the other sex.

Generalized amnesia   Failure to recall one's entire life.

Generalized anxiety disorder   Chronic (at least six months), generalized, and persistent anxiety without the specific symptoms that characterize phobic disorders, panic disorders, or obsessive compulsive disorders.

Genital phase   The final stage of psychosexual development.

Globus hystericus   Sensation of a lump in the throat.

Grandiose delusions   An exaggerated belief in one's own importance.

Grief (bereavement)   A normal, appropriate, affective sadness in response to a recognizable external loss.

Group psychotherapy   Application of psychotherapeutic techniques to a group, including utilization of interactions of members of the group.

Hallucinations   False sensory perceptions that are not caused by external stimuli.

Histrionic personality disorder (hysterical personality)   A disorder showing a pattern of theatrical behavior that is overly reactive, intensely expressed, and perceived by others as shallow, superficial, or insincere; interpersonal relationships are characteristically redistrubed, and sexual adjustment is poor.

Holism   The understanding of the individual personality based on the interplay of one's inherited structure, one's uniqueness, and the cultural pattern in which one lives.

Homeostasis   The individual's tendency to maintain a relatively stable psychological condition with respect to contending drives, motivations, and other psychodynamic forces.

Hostile identification   Internalization of undesirable personality traits of parent or authority figures.

Hostility   Anger, antagonism, opposition, or resistance in thought or behavior.

Humanistic therapies   A number of therapeutic approaches characterized by their phenomenological or existential assumptions about human experiences and/or by their opposition to traditional psychoanalysis or behavior therapy.

Huntington's chorea   A degenerative disease of the basal ganglia and cerebral cortex.

Hypermnesia   Abnormally vivid or complete memory, or the reawakening of impressions long seemingly forgotten.

Hypersomnia   Excessive sleep.

Hypertension (essential)   A systemic reaction in which there is a sustained elevation of blood pressure above 140/90 in the absence of any demonstrable pathology.

Hyperventilation syndrome   A condition in which the individual is subject to repeated forced respirations, yawning, sensations of hunger for air, occasional tetany, chest pain, lightheadedness, paresthesias of the hand, feet, and face, and an intense conviction of impending death.

Hypnagogic hallucinations (hypnagogic imagery)   Mental images that sometimes occur just before sleep.

Hypnopompic hallucinations   Images seen in dreams that persist after awakening.

Hypnotherapy   The use of hypnosis as a means of facilitating psychotherapy.

Hypochondriasis   An unrealistic interpretation of physical signs or sensations as abnormal, leading to the preoccupation with the fear of having a disease or belief that one already has one.

Hypomania (mild mania)   Characterized by increased happiness or optimism.

Id   The unconscious reservoir of primitive drives (instincts).

Idealization   The overestimation of admired qualities of another person or desired object.

Idealized self   A glorified self-image, closely related to the current concepts of narcissism; a sign of neurosis.

Ideational depressions   Depressed mental content with few, if any, physical or motor symptoms.

Identification   The unconscious, wishful adoption or internalization of the personality characteristics or identity of another individual, generally one possessing attributes that the subject envies or admires.

Identification with the aggressor   The unconscious internalization of the characteristics of a frustrating or feared person (may be parent or parent substitute).

Identity   An inner sense of sameness that perseveres, despite external changes.

Illusions   Misinterpretation of sensory experiences, usually optical or auditory.

Imitation   Conscious mimicking of the behavior of others.

Inappropriateness   An affect opposite to what would be expected.

Incest   Sexual relations between members of the same family (e.g., parent-child, brother-sister).

Incoherence   Disorderly, illogical thought, sometimes manifested as garbled speech.

Incorporation   A primitive defense mechanism in which the psychic image of another person is wholly or partially assimilated into an individual's personality.

Increased attention (hyperprosexia)   Unusual attention, usually to details of personal significance.

Inferiority complex   The conflict, partly conscious and partly unconscious, that impels the individual to attempt to overcome the distress accompanying feelings of inferiority.

Influential delusions   The belief that one can control or be controlled by another's behavior or thoughts; most commonly observed in paranoid or schizophrenic disorders.

Intellectualization   The overuse of intellectual concepts and words to avoid feeling or expressing of emotion.

Interest tests   Tests that compare the individual response patterns with the response patterns of persons representative of a number of professions and occupations.

Intermittent explosive disorder   A disorder in which individuals have recurrent and paroxysmal episodes of significant loss of control of aggressive impulses that result in serious assault of destruction of property.

Intoxication syndrome   Recent ingestion and presence in the body of a toxic substance in which there is maladaptive behavior during the waking state due to the effect of the substance on the central nervous system.

Intrapsychic   That which occurs within the personality.

Introjection   The symbolic internalization or assimilation (taking into oneself) of a loved or hated person or external object.

Introversion   Inwardly directed libido, reflected in the tendency to be preoccupied with oneself.

Involutional melancholia   A psychotic reaction with initial onset in the involutional period (late middle life), most commonly characterized by depressive affect but occasionally by paranoid mentation.

Irrelevance   Thinking that is erroneous or irrelevant to the subject at hand.

Irritable bowel   A functional bowel disorder characterized by periods of diarrhea, alternating with periods of constipation, abdominal cramps, flatulence, and sometimes by increased mucus in the stool.

Isolated explosive disorder   A disorder in which individuals have had a single discrete episode, characterized by failure to resist an impulse that led to a single violent, externally directed act, which had catastrophic impact on others, and for which the available information does not justify the diagnosis of schizophrenia, antisocial personality disorder, or conduct disorder.

Isolation   The separation of an unacceptable impulse, act, or idea from its memory origin, thereby removing the emotional charge associated with the original memory.

Jamais vu   A false feeling of unfamiliarity with a real situation one has experienced before.

Kleptomania   A disorder in which there is a recurrent failure to resist impulses to steal objects, not for immediate use or their monetary value.

Korsakoff's syndrome   Alcohol amnestic syndrome. *See* Amnestic syndrome.

La belle indifference   Indifference to an illness.

Latency   The stage between the oedipal period and the adolescent years.

Latent homosexuality   Homosexual desires that are largely unconscious, unrecognized, and projected or sublimated.

Libido   The emotional energy broadly derived from the underlying instincts (psychosexual energy) and presumably present at birth.

Libido development   Stages of psychosexual development.

Lithium   A salt used in the treatment of psychotic excitements, especially elated episodes.

Localized amnesia   Failure to recall all events during a circumscribed period of time.

Logorrhea (volubility)   Uncontrollable, rapid, excessive talking.

Macropsia   Visualization of objects as being larger than they really are.

Magical thinking   The imputation of reality to a thought.

Malingering   Conscious simulation of illness in order to avoid an unpleasant or intolerable alternative.

Management therapy   Activities apart from formal psychotherapy, group psychotherapy, somatic therapy, or electroconvulsive therapy, and chemotherapy that have psychotherapeutic value.

Mania   Mental state characterized by flight of ideas, elated or grandiose mood, and psychomotor excitement (generalized physical and emotional overactivity).

Mannerisms   Stereotyped movements such as blinking, grimacing, gesturing.

Masculine protest   The term for the individual's attempt to escape from the feminine, submissive role.

Megalomania   Pathological preoccupation with delusions of omnipotence or wealth.

Mental status examination   A special form of assessment, often conducted in conjunction with the history-taking interview.

Methadone substitution   Approach in which addict takes a regular dose of methadone, given orally, after which the addict is progressively withdrawn from the drug over a period of a few days.

Micropsia   Visualization of objects as being smaller than they really are.

Migraine headaches   A syndrome characterized by recurrent, severe unilateral headache (cephalgia), nausea, vomiting, and certain prodromal (for which previous warning has been given) disturbances (scotoma, paresthesia or speech difficulty).

Minnesota Multiphasic Personality Inventory   The most widely used objective personality test in psychiatric practice in the United States; consists of 550 true-false items.

Misidentification   Incorrect identification of other people.

Monozygotic twins   Identical twins.

Moral masochism   The seeking of humiliation and failure, as opposed to physical pain.

Multiple personality   The domination of the individual by one of two or more distinct personalities at any one time.

Mutism   A form of negativism characterized by refusal to speak, for conscious or unconscious reasons.

Narcissistic personality disorder   A personality disorder in which the features are a grandiose sense of self-importance or uniqueness; preoccupation with fantasies of unlimited success; exhibitionistic need for constant attention and admiration; characteristic responses to threats to self-esteem; characteristic disturbances in interpersonal relationships, such as lack of empathy, entitlement, interpersonal exploitiveness, and relationships that vacillate between the extremes of over-idealization and devaluation.

Narcissistic or pregenital phase   The oral and anal phases considered together.

Necrophilia   The deriving of sexual gratification from corpses.

Negative reinforcement   The termination of a noxious or aversive stimulus.

Negativism   Opposition, resistance, or refusal to accept reasonable suggestions or advice; a tendency to be in opposition.

Neologism   A coined word or condensation of several words to express a complex idea.

Neuromodulators   Act to amplify or dampen the degree and duration of neurotransmitter action, providing for a "fine tuning" of nervous system activity.

Neurosis   A term formerly used to describe maladaptive emotional states resulting from unresolved unconscious conflicts (in general, not used in *DSM-III*).

Neurotransmitters   Act at the synapses where communication among neurons occurs.

Nihilistic delusions   The belief that oneself, the environment, or the world does not exist.

Nocturnal anxiety   The infant's fear of the dark.

Object libido   Libido that is directed outward toward another person or thing.

Objective test   Test that is scored in a standardized way; the results are expressed in numerical scores.

Obsessions   Recurrent and persistent ideas, thoughts, or impulses that are ego dystonic; that is, they are not experienced as voluntarily produced, but rather as ideas that invade the consciousness and are experienced as senseless or repugnant.

Obsessive-compulsive disorder   Recurrent obsessions or compulsions or both of these.

Occupational therapy   The utilization of activities and situations psychotherapeutically to meet the individual's needs and provide a vehicle for personal change and growth.

Oedipus complex   The attachment of the child for the parent of the opposite sex, accompanied by envious and aggressive feelings toward the parent of the same sex.

Oral phase   The first twelve to eighteen months of life, characterized chiefly by preoccupation with feeding.

Oral-sadistic phase   The later oral phase, or biting stage, that is aggressive.

Organic mental disorder   A disorder in which there is transient or permanent dysfunction of the brain attributed to specific organic factors judged to be necessary to the disturbance.

Orgasm phase   The peaking of sexual pleasure accompanied by rhythmic contraction of the perineal muscles and pelvic reproductive organs and release of sexual tension.

Orientation   Awareness of one's relationship to time, surroundings, and other persons.

Overcompensation   An exaggerated attempt at overcoming inferiorities.

Panic   An acute anxiety attack of overwhelming severity that leads to disorganization of ego functions.

Panic disorders   Recurrent panic (anxiety) attacks and nervousness.

Paramnesia   Distortion or falsification of memory in which the individual confuses reality and fantasy.

Paranoia   A psychotic disorder characterized by an elaborate, well-systematized, complex, intricate, logical, and well-fixed single delusional system, and relatively good preservation of the remainder of the personality.

Paranoid disorders   Psychotic disorders in which the predominant symptoms are delusions, generally persecutory, jealous, or grandiose. They usually are without hallucinations and cannot be explained by other psychotic disorders in which paranoid symptoms may be prominent.

Paranoid personality   A personality disorder exhibiting a pervasive and long-standing suspiciousness and mistrust of people, hypersensitivity, hypervigilance, unwarranted suspicion, jealousy, envy, excessive self-importance, and a tendency to blame others and ascribe evil motives to them.

Paraphilia   A disorder characterized by sexual arousal in response to objects or situations that are not normally arousing and by gross impairment of the capacity for affectionate sexual activity with human partners.

Paraphrenia   A disorder characterized by paranoid delusions without deterioration, dementia, or loss of contact with reality other than in the area of the delusional system.

Paresis   Muscular weakness.

Partialism   Preoccupation with certain parts of the female body.

Passive-aggressive personality disorder   A disorder in which there is resistance to demands for adequate activity or performance in both occupational and social functioning that is not expressed directly; as a consequence, there is pervasive and long-standing social or occupational ineffectiveness.

Passive influence   The psychotic belief that one is being controlled by others.

Pathological gambling   A disorder with features of chronic and progressive preoccupation with gambling and the urge to gamble; gambling behavior that compromises, disrupts, or damages personal, family, and/or vocational pursuits.

Pedophilia   A disorder in which there is preference for repetitive sexual activity with prepubertal children of either sex.

Penis envy   The girl's desire to possess a penis and thus to be masculine.

Perception   The awareness and intended integration of sensory impressions of the environment and their interpretation in light of experience.

Periodic catatonia   A rare form of episodic catatonia that is related to shifts in the individual's metabolic nitrogen balance.

Persecutory delusions   A belief that one is singled out for oppression, attack, or harassment.

Perseveration   A persistent, repetitive expression of a single idea in response to various questions.

Persona   The social facade assumed by an individual (so named from the mask worn by actors in ancient Greek drama that characterized the mood portrayed).

Personality   The sum total of a person's internal and external patterns of adjustment to life.

Personality disorders   Disorders characterized by deeply ingrained, inflexible, maladaptive patterns of relating to, perceiving, and thinking about the environment and oneself that are of sufficient severity to cause either significant impairment in adaptive functioning or subjective distress.

Persuasion   Direct suggestion, inducement, or entreatment in an effort to influence a patient's behavior.

Phallic stage   Period extending from the end of the third year to the seventh year.

Pharmacotherapy (chemotherapy)   The treatment of psychiatric disorders with drugs.

Phenothiazines   Drugs used in treating schizophrenic symptoms that act to inhibit or block dopamine-mediated transmission.

Pregenital phase   The oral and anal phases considered together.

Primary processes   The psychological expressions of the underlying basic drives.

Primordial images   A phylogenetic memory, heavily laden with mythological reference.

Projection   The attributing to another person or object, thoughts, feelings, motives, or desires that are really one's own disavowed and unacceptable traits.

Projective identification   The association of uncomfortable aspects of one's own personality, with their projection onto another person, resulting in identification with the other person.

Psychoanalysis   A collection of data based on observations that lead to a theory of abnormal behavior as well as to a general theory of normal personality development; the name of a psychotherapeutic technique.

Psychoanalytic therapy   The exploration of the unconscious, chiefly through free association.

Psychobiological therapy   Critical examination and evaluation of conscious forces in the patient's personality development and emotional problems (that is, the patient attempts to consciously analyze and to synthesize).

Psychobiology   Adolf Meyer's psychiatric theory that "studies not only the person as a whole, as a unit, but also the whole man."

Psychodrama   A form of therapy in which the patients dramatize their emotional problems in a group setting.

Psychodynamics   The study, explanation, or interpretation of behavior or mental states in terms of mental or emotional forces or processes.

Psychogenic amnesia   A sudden onset of a disturbance in the ability to recall important personal information registered and stored in memory, in the absence of an underlying organic mental disorder; the travelling to another locale with the assumption of a new identity.

Psychogenic fugue   The sudden unexpected departure from home or customary work locale and the assumption of a new identity but retaining the ability to recall one's prior identity, in the absence of an underlying organic mental disorder.

Psychogenic pain disorder (psychalgia)   A clinical picture in which the predominant disturbance is pain (usually severe and prolonged) in the absence of adequate physical findings, not attributable to any other mental or physical disorder or out of proportion to the physical findings and associated with evidence of psychological etiology.

Psychomotor excitement   Mentally and physically hyperactive response to internal or external stimuli.

Psychomotor retardation   The slowing down of mental and physical activity.

Psychophysiological disorders   Those physical conditions either with demonstrable organic pathology (such as rheumatoid arthritis) or a known pathophysiological process (such as migraine headaches) that show evidence of temporal relationship to psychologically meaningful environmental stimuli in the initiation, exacerbation, or maintenance of the physical symptoms.

Psychosexual dysfunctions   Inhibitions of the appetitive or psychophysiological changes that characterize the sexual response cycle.

Psychosocial stressors   Usual stresses of life.

Psychosomatic reactions   *See* Psychophysiological disorders.

Psychosurgery   A group of various surgical procedures that have been developed and are directed at selected areas of the brain, depending upon the type of disabling symptoms present.

Psychotherapy   A process in which a person who wishes to change symptoms or problems in living or is seeking personal growth enters, implicitly or explicitly, into a contract to interact in a prescribed way with a psychotherapist.

Psychotic depression   Depression so profound that the patient loses contact with reality, develops delusions, and frequently is a serious suicidal risk.

Pyromania   A disorder in which there is recurrent failure to resist impulses to set fires and the intense fascination with the setting of fires and seeing fires burn.

Rapport   The feeling of harmonious accord, mutual responsiveness, and sympathy that contributes to the patient's confidence in the therapist and willingness to work cooperatively with him or her.

Rationalization   The ascribing of acceptable or worthwhile motives to one's own thoughts, feelings, or behavior that really have unrecognized motives.

Reaction formation   The direction of overt behavior or attitudes in precisely the opposite direction of the individual's underlying, unacceptable conscious or unconscious impulses.

Reactive drinking   The type of drinking that is done in response to some particular emotional stress as, for example, the death of a loved one.

Real self   The unique total force and sense of integration found in each person.

Reassurance   The imparting or restoration of confidence and freeing the patient from fear and anxiety.

Recall   The ability to recount a registered experience.

Referential delusion   The belief that the irrelevant remarks or acts of others refers to oneself.

Registration   The ability to establish a record of an experience in the central nervous system.

Regression   The unconscious return to an earlier level of emotional adjustment at which gratification was assured.

Repression   The involuntary, automatic banishment of unacceptable ideas, impulses, or feelings into the unconscious (motivated unconscious forgetting).

Reserpine   A drug that depletes levels of serotonin, norepinephrine, and dopamine in patients and in some cases produces an accompanying clinical depression.

Resistance   The conscious or unconscious psychological forces in the patient that oppose bringing repressed (unconscious) material into consciousness.

Resolution   A sense of well-being and general relaxation.

Restitution   The supplanting of a highly valued object that has been lost through rejection by, or death or departure of, another object.

Retention   The persistence or permanence of a registered experience.

Retrospective falsification   The unconscious distortion of past experiences to conform to present emotional needs.

Rorschach test   The best-known and most widely used of the projective techniques, with materials consisting of ten ink blots.

Sado-masochism   The occurrence of both sadism and masochism in the same person.

Schizoaffective disorder   A depressive or manic *syndrome* that precedes or develops concurrently with psychotic *symptoms* incompatible with an affective disorder. Includes some *symptoms* characteristic of *schizophrenia* and other symptoms seen in *major affective disorders.*[1]

Schizoid personality (introverted personality)   A disorder characterized by a defect in the capacity to form social relationships; introversion and bland or constricted affect.

Schizophrenic disorders   A large group of disorders usually of psychotic proportion, manifested by characteristic disturbances of language and communication, thought, perception, affect, and behavior that lasts longer than six months. Thought disturbances are marked by alterations of concept formation that may lead to misinterpretation of reality, misperceptions, and sometimes delusions and hallucinations.

Schizophreniform disorder   A disorder in which the features are identical to those of schizophrenia, with the exception that the duration is less than six months, but more than one week.

Schizotypal personality   A disorder with various oddities of thinking, perception, communication, and behavior, but never severe enough to meet the criteria for schizophrenia.

Secondary affective disorders   Disorder occurring in persons who have had other psychiatric illnesses (e.g., schizophrenia or alcoholism) or who have suffered an affective disorder related to a medical condition.

Secondary processes   Reasonable and acceptable ways in which the underlying basic drives are controlled and permitted expression according to the demands of the outside world.

Selective amnesia   Failure to recall some but not all of the events that occurred during a circumscribed period of time.

Self-accusatory delusion   The belief that one is responsible for harm.

Self-help groups   Groups without professionally trained leaders in which the group experience does not uncover basic conflicts, but does offer new shared experiences to the patient.

Self-regulation techniques   Techniques in which a person learns to discriminate the environmental settings for maladaptive behaviors and to manage one's own reinforcing consequences.

Senium   The geriatric age; the period of old age.

Separation anxiety   Apprehension noted in infants when they are removed from their mothers or mother surrogates.

Sexual masochism   A disorder in which sexual excitement is produced in an individual by his or her own suffering.

Sexual sadism   A disorder in which the essential feature is inflicting physical or psychological suffering on another person as a method of stimulating sexual excitement and orgasm, during which there are insistent and persistent fantasies in which sexual excitement is produced as a result of suffering inflicted on the partner.

Shared paranoid disorder (folie à deux)   A psychotic disorder in which two closely related people, usually members of the same family and who live in close and intimate association, share identical delusions.

Simple phobia   A persistent, irrational fear of public places, being away from home, or of humiliation or embarrassment, and a compelling desire to avoid an object or a situation other than being alone.

Social phobia   A persistent, irrational fear of and compelling desire to avoid a situation in which the individual is exposed to possible scrutiny by others and fears that he or she may act in a way that may be humiliating.

Somatic delusion   A deluded interpretation of physical symptoms.

Somatic (motor visceral) manifestations   The resultant of the physiological responses of the various bodily systems to the increased secretion of epinephrine.

Somatization disorder (Briquet's syndrome)   Recurrent and multiple somatic complaints for which medical attention is sought but that are not apparently due to any physical disorder.

Somatoform disorders   A group of disorders with physical symptoms suggestive of physical disorders for which there is no demonstrable findings or known physiological mechanism, but instead, positive evidence of a strong presumption that the symptoms are linked to psychological factors or conflicts.

Somnambulism   Sleep walking.

Splitting   The inability to unite and integrate the hating and loving aspects of both one's self-image and one's image of another person.

Stereotypy   The persistent repetition of a motor activity.

Stranger anxiety   The apprehension noted in infants when approached by strangers.

Sublimation   The diversion of unacceptable, instinctual drives into socially sanctioned channels.

Substitution   An unconscious replacement of a highly valued but unattainable or unacceptable emotional goal or object by one which is attainable or acceptable.

Successful defenses   Defenses that eliminate the need for immediate gratification or provide substitute, socially acceptable gratification.

Succinylcholine chloride (Anectine)   A drug used to modify the muscular contractions of the convulsive seizures.

Superego   The censoring force of the personality.

Supportive psychotherapy   The form of psychotherapy that deals predominantly with conscious material and is centered chiefly on support of the individual's strength and assets.

Suppression   The voluntary, intentional relegation of unacceptable ideas or impulses to the foreconscious (volitional exclusion or conscious forgetting).

Symbolization   The unconscious mechanism by which a neutral idea or object is used to represent another idea or object that has a forbidden aspect.

Symptomatic alcoholism   Condition in which drinking is a symptom of a serious emotional disorder, such as anxiety disorder, affective disorder, or schizophrenic disorder.

Tangentiality   Inability to reach the thinking goal.

Telephone scatologia (lewdness)   A disorder in which sexual gratification is derived, usually by men who telephone women, make obscene remarks, and suggest that the woman should meet them and engage in sexual activity.

Tension   Tautness, motor and emotional restlessness; dread.

Test   A systematic procedure of obtaining samples of behavior for the comparison of two or more persons.

Thanatos   The term for the aggressive, destructive, or death forces.

Thematic Apperception Test (TAT)   A test consisting of twenty illustrations. The patient is asked to tell a story about the content of each picture.

Therapeutic reaction   The use of recreational activities therapeutically to promote personal change and growth.

Thinking   The exercising of powers of judgment, conception, or inference as distinguished from simple sensory perception.

Thought broadcasting   The belief that the individual's thoughts are broadcasts from his or her head into the external world.

Thought insertion   The insertion of thoughts that are not one's own into one's mind.

Thought withdrawal   The withdrawal of thoughts from one's head; delusions of being controlled or delusions of passivity (that feelings, impulses, thoughts, or actions are not one's own and are imposed on one by some external force.)

Tolerance   Condition in which repeated equal doses have a diminishing effect (more and more of the drug is needed to produce the effect produced by the first use).

Toxic deliria   Substance-induced syndrome.

Trance state   A psychological stupor characterized by immobility and unresponsiveness to the environment.

Transference   The displacement of feelings for significant people in one's earlier life onto the physician or therapist.

Transsexualism   A disorder in which there is a persistent sense of discomfort and inappropriateness about one's anatomic sex and a persistent wish to be rid of one's genitals and to live as a member of the opposite sex.

Transvestitism   A disorder in which there is sexual arousal from wearing the clothes of the opposite sex.

Tricyclics   Drugs that block the reuptake of biogenic amine neurotransmitters from synapses, thus increasing the concentration of the neurotransmitters in the synapse.

Ulcerative colitis   An acute and chronic disease of the mucosa and submucosa of the colon.

Unburdening (ventilation; catharsis)   The therapeutic release of feelings through conscious, free expression.

Unconscious   That part of the mind that is made up of drives, feelings, ideas, and urges that are outside the individual's awareness.

Uncovering therapy (intensive psychotherapy, insight psychotherapy, investigative therapy)   Therapy whose aim it is to produce insight by uncovering conflicts, chiefly unconscious, so they can be dealt with more effectively.

Undoing   A primitive defense mechanism in which some unacceptable past behavior is symbolically acted out in reverse, usually repetitiously (symbolic atonement).

Unsuccessful defenses   Defenses that do not resolve the conflict and the continuing need for the defense.

Uralagnia   The desire to urinate on a sexual partner or to be urinated upon.

Vasodepressor syncope   A fainting due to acute peripheral circulatory inadequacy (with a sudden drop in blood pressure) that is quickly reversible.

Verbigeration   The meaningless repetition of incoherent words or sentences.

Voyeurism   A disorder in which there is repetitive seeking out of situations in which the individual engages in looking at unsuspecting women who are either naked, in the act of disrobing, or engaging in sexual activity.

Waxyflexibility (cerea flexibilitas)   A condition in which a patient passively retains the position into which he or she has been placed.

Wernicke's syndrome   A rare disorder of central nervous system metabolism, associated with a thiamine deficiency and seen chiefly in chronic alcoholics.

Withdrawal   A substance-specific syndrome that follows the cessation or reduction of the intake of a substance.

Word-salad   An incomprehensible and incoherent mixture of words and phrases.

Zoophilia (bestiality)   A disorder in which there is use of animals as the preferred or exclusive method of producing sexual excitement.

Index

MMPI, 251
Monozygotic twins, 200, 211
Moral masochism, 154
Morel, Benedict Augustin, 208
Mowrer, O.H., 279
Multiple personality, 96
Münchausen syndrome, 102
Mutism, 40
Mydriasis, 46

Narcissism
    primary, 13
Narcissistic phase, 14
Necrophilia, 157
Negativism, 40
Neologism, 39
Neurocirculatory asthenia (NCA), 114
Neuroendocrine, 45
Neurotic characters, 136
Neurotics
    acting out, 136
Nonsense syndrome, 102

Obesity, 108
Objective psyche, 17
Obsessions, 36, 76
Obsessive-compulsive disorder, 76
Obsessive-compulsive neurosis, 76
Obsessive-ruminative state, 77
Oedipus complex, 15
Operant conditioning, 26
Opioid substances, 165
Oral phase, 14
Oral-sadistic, 14
Organic
    brain syndrome, 236, 237
    mental disorders, 236, 237
Orgasm, 159
Orientation, 34
Overcompensation, 57

Panic, 31
    disorders, 73
Paramnesia, 33
Paranoia, 228
Paranoid condition, 230
Paranoid disorders, 226
    atypical, 230
    other, 230
    shared, 231
Paranoid jealousy, 228
Paranoid state, 230
Paraphilias, 142
Paraphrenia, 230
Paresis, 87
Partialism, 147
Pathological gambling, 136
Pavlov, Ivan, 24, 279

Pedophilia, 150
Penis envy, 15
Peptic ulcer, 110
Perception, 34
Perls, Fritz, 284
Perseveration, 38
Persona, 17
Personality, 10, 118
    anancastic, 78, 131
    hysterical, 122
    interpersonal theory of, 19
    introverted, 121
    paranoid, 120
    premorbid, 78
    psychopathic, 124
    schizoid, 121
    schizotypal, 121
Personality disorders, 118
    antisocial, 124, 136
    avoidant, 130
    borderline, 129
    compulsive, 131
    dependent, 130
    histrionic, 122
    narcissistic, 123
    passive-aggressive, 132
Persuasion, 266
Phallic phase, 14
Pharmacotherapy, 271
Phencyclidine, 167
Phobias, 36, 69
    simple, 71
    social, 70
Phobic
    disorders, 68
    neurosis, 68
    reaction, 68
Photographic memory, 36
Pleasure principle, 11
Polatin, P., 208
Porphyria, 3
Post-traumatic stress disorder, 80
    chronic, 80
Posturizing, 40
Preconscious, 12
Pregenital phase, 14
Preoccupations, 36, 40
Pressure of speech, 39
Primordial images, 17
Projection, 55
Pseudoneurological symptoms, 84
Psychalgia, 90
Psychoanalysis, 11
    existential, 22
Psychobiology, 21
Psychodrama, 276
Psychodynamics, 10